All THE BEST,

[signature]

```
D1265478
```

PRAISE FOR *FINDING HEART IN ART*

"*This powerful exposition daringly reveals the struggle of an erudite healer proficient in helping others but ill-equipped to save himself. In his own journey of self-discovery, not unlike the conversion of Ignatius de Loyola, Shawn experienced a transformative epiphany that restored to him a life nearly lost. As an emergency physician reflecting upon my own experience, Shawn's story strikes painfully close to home. In this time of growing clinician disillusionment and burnout, this timely work is valuable both to healers seeking their own journeys of redemption and their family, friends, and patients who love and rely upon them.*"

—Steven J. Stack, MD

ER physician, Lexington, KY

"Finding Heart in Art *is more than a book; it is a channel of grace that may save your life. For those experiencing burnout or a numbness to life, rediscover what it means to connect with yourself, to be human made in the image of God, and to embrace beauty, creativity, and imagination all over again. Dr. Shawn Jones has provided a map for your journey filled with personal stories, captivating art, solid research, and exercises for reflection. Come and be transformed.*"

—Zach Fay

CEO and creator of Lightgliders, St. Louis, MO

FINDING HEART
IN ART

FINDING HEART
IN ART

A SURGEON'S RENAISSANCE APPROACH TO HEALING MODERN MEDICAL BURNOUT

SHAWN C. JONES, MD, FACS

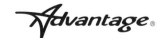

Published by Advantage, Charleston, South Carolina.
Member of Advantage Media Group.

ADVANTAGE is a registered trademark, and the Advantage colophon is a trademark of Advantage Media Group, Inc.

Printed in the United States of America.

10 9 8 7 6 5 4 3 2 1

ISBN: 978-1-59932-866-9
LCCN: 2017958770

Cover design by Carly Blake.
Layout design by Megan Elger.

This publication is designed to provide accurate and authoritative information in regard to the subject matter covered. It is sold with the understanding that the publisher is not engaged in rendering legal, accounting, or other professional services. If legal advice or other expert assistance is required, the services of a competent professional person should be sought.

Advantage Media Group is proud to be a part of the Tree Neutral® program. Tree Neutral offsets the number of trees consumed in the production and printing of this book by taking proactive steps such as planting trees in direct proportion to the number of trees used to print books. To learn more about Tree Neutral, please visit **www.treeneutral.com**.

Advantage Media Group is a publisher of business, self-improvement, and professional development books. We help entrepreneurs, business leaders, and professionals share their Stories, Passion, and Knowledge to help others Learn & Grow. Do you have a manuscript or book idea that you would like us to consider for publishing? Please visit **advantagefamily.com** or call **1.866.775.1696**.

To Evelyn

DISCLAIMER

In order to protect privacy, all patient names have been changed. Other identifying characteristics have additionally been changed. Doctors are not identified by their real names in some instances.

TABLE OF CONTENTS

ABOUT THE AUTHOR

Dr. Shawn Jones is a board-certified otolaryngologist-head and neck surgeon who is trained in minimally invasive robotic surgery. He is the senior and founding member of his specialty group, Purchase ENT, which he began in 1995. Dr. Jones lives in Paducah, Kentucky, with his wife Evelyn, who is a practicing dermatologist. They have three adult children. Dr. Evelyn and Dr. Shawn are both active in their church where he serves as an elder.

Dr. Jones was president of the Kentucky Medical Association (KMA) from 2011 to 2012, after serving on the board of trustees for over fifteen years. In 2016 he was honored with the association's Distinguished Service Award. He serves on KMA's American Medical Association delegation and was recently elected president of the Kentucky Foundation for Medical Care. He also is a member of the gratis faculty of the University of Louisville School of Medicine in the Department of Otolaryngology.

Dr. Jones is a public health advocate who championed a local smoke-free ordinance in Paducah. He has appeared on Kentucky Educational Television numerous times in support of a smoke-free Kentucky. He also regularly uses his expertise to help the under-served on medical mission trips, previously traveling to Romania, Kenya, and Honduras. An avid reader and scholar, Dr. Jones enjoys biographies and history books, biblical commentaries, and books on spirituality.

ACKNOWLEDGMENTS

My deepest thanks to those who helped me on this journey:

Evelyn, Rebecca, Shawn Jr., and Caleb. My father, Bill. My mother, Linda, who died last year. Stephen, Chip, Phil, Dane, David and all the "glad men" with me in the meat grinder at the CPE. The Monday night group—you know who you are. Regina, Scott, Corie, Laura, Wes, and especially Rusty Shelton, along with everyone else at Advantage Media Group | Forbes Books. Lisa Tener, Jacqueline Wehmueller, John Hanc, Julie Silver, and the Harvard Writers Conference attendees over the last two years for the encouragement, feedback, and direction. Kelly Walden for graciously reviewing the entire manuscript. Dr. Buddy Payne, Ben Hall, Dan Lankford, and F. Lagard Smith for the chapter reviews, criticism, help with exegesis, advice, rebuke, dire predictions of failure, stimulation and inspiration. I am indebted.

INTRODUCTION

Dwell on the past and you'll lose an eye.
Forget the past and you'll lose both eyes.

—Aleksandr Solzhenitsyn

Finding Heart in Art is a personal story about the journey to recover my heart, which I neglected and nearly lost during my training as a medical student, as a resident, and during my early years as a surgeon. My story is a metaphoric, Homeric odyssey—a journey home through tempestuous waters fraught with trials, a journey that traverses the most foreboding geography in existence: the distance that lies between a man's head and his heart.

The noted writer Erma Bombeck once said, "It takes a lot of courage to show your dreams to someone else." What, then, does it take to show someone your nightmares? I asked myself that question frequently while writing this book. Along the way, I also discovered that telling the story of my nightmarish journey must be coupled with purpose. Otherwise, the admission risks a lapse into tawdry exhibitionism.

I'm telling my story in hopes that it will serve as a roadmap to recovery for others, and maybe even keep them from abandoning their heart in the first place. Nearly all of us lose a part of ourselves and, at some point, have to travel to find that which has been lost. The details of our journeys differ, but we all have a homecoming we seek.

Addressing and healing my own wounds were achieved, in part, by recognizing the beauty in art, specifically through a smattering of the best paintings and artists of the Renaissance. These pieces detail my journey of healing from beginning to end and, naturally, follow my career as a physician. I chose the works because of how they moved me and because of the emotions they stirred within me, not just because of the stories they told and the truth they reflected on my life as a doctor. Like opening a wound and allowing it to heal from the inside out, discovering my emotions through these paintings was painful, but it was also healing. Medical training can desensitize one over time, dehumanizing you in a way that is similar to the effects of post-traumatic stress disorder (PTSD). Surgeons in particular have a tendency to put emotions in a box and set them aside—something their medical training teaches very well.

Reconnecting with beauty through art, music, or similar therapies is a common treatment for people suffering from trauma. It can be a means of expressing the truth of emotions that are difficult to handle, as well as a way of reanimating life through an appreciation of something outside the self. Research indicates that creativity is associated with improved emotional functioning.[1] Multiple studies show that engaging in the creative arts can lower stress and anxiety and improve mood. Some studies demonstrate that forty-five minutes of art therapy can lead to a reduction in cortisol levels. One study even finds that creativity and imagination can help people identify their "reservoir of healing;" the more we understand the relationship

---

1   Tamlin S. Conner, Colin G. DeYoung, and Paul J. Silvia, "Everyday Creative Activity as a Path to Flourishing," *The Journal of Positive Psychology* (November 2016), http://dx.doi.org/10.1080/17439760.2016.1257049.

between creative expression and healing, the more we will discover the healing power of the arts.[2]

My journey is one of finding access to my emotional nature by reconnecting with beauty, through which I discovered I was able to find and name my emotions. I was able to experience—from the heart—gladness, hurt, loneliness, sadness, anger, fear, guilt, and shame.[3] These emotions are the voice of my heart, and express the truth of who I am. Similarly, your feelings, longings, desires, and needs as a human being are a reflection of who you are. They will have their say, one way or another.

My book is not only about the healing journey and how an individual can respond to their emotions, but it's also about looking at the workplace and finding ways to facilitate structural change within organizations to promote wellness and healing. With so many physicians experiencing burnout, what can be done to alter the system?

2   Heather Stuckey and Jeremy Nobel, "The Connection between Art, Healing and Public Health: A Review of Current Literature," *American Journal of Public Health* 100, no. 2 (February 2010): 254–263.

3   Chip Dodd, *The Voice of the Heart: A Call to Full Living,* 2nd ed. (Nashville: Sage Hill Resources, 2014), 135.

ONE

MY FALL AND REDEMPTION

There is a road from the eye to the heart that does not go through the intellect.

—G. K. Chesterton

I am a surgeon. I am used to creating wounds, identifying wounds, treating wounds, and watching them heal. For over twenty years I practiced my craft, acquiring the skills, knowledge, and wisdom necessary to do so adeptly. Imagine my dismay when I recognized I had my own deep emotional wounds that had not healed, because—at least in part—I had never looked at them. I eventually reached a point where it became necessary to lay aside my scalpel and address my needs as a human being. I braved my own disapprobation to do so.

A pivotal point in my journey occurred when I woke up one morning and realized I wasn't "feeling" anything. I recall staring at my reflection in the mirror wondering what was going on. I could still "feel" in the tactile sense; I was able to shave and dress and get on with my day. But there was a significant emotional numbness. Even worse, I approached the dilemma as if I were an unimpassioned observer. That's when terror began to creep in. I was experiencing alexithymia and was completely unable to identify or feel anything in the way of happiness or sadness, anger, or calm. I felt no connection to anything—myself, my family, my associates, my patients. I felt completely disconnected from the world around me.

In retrospect, my experience was not so much an explosion nor a burnout as it was the result of a very slow leak punctuated by multiple traumatic episodes. Some of these were self-inflicted and some were perpetrated, but there was no single event that sent me over the edge. There have been multiple places in my life where a change might have interrupted the course of events that led to me being in this state of mind. But instead of stepping back and slowing down, I began to work harder—just as I was trained to do. When I felt some unease with my professional satisfaction, I wondered if I might want to do something different as a career. What's crazy is that I knew, deep down, that a major part of me simply loved being a physician, and doing the work of a physician. I loved operating. In my search for peace regarding my condition, I did what I knew to do. As a workaholic on steroids would do, I added more cases. I stayed up later. I read more. I started working on a master's degree in business administration. I just added things, which hastened my demise.

Physicians see a lot of ugliness every day, to the point that it doesn't bother them. Our world—in which the body is opened, broken, fractured—is not the normal human experience. Even though we are repairing it, fixing it, helping it, we see things that cause most people to pass out, be repulsed, or at least look away. We deal with disease, death, dismemberment, suffering, loss, and heartache on a daily basis.

However, some days are worse than others. By chance and circumstance I have cared for some patients struck by unusually savage senselessness: the Carrolton bus tragedy in which a bus carrying members of a church youth group was struck head on by a pickup truck driven by an inebriated man and traveling the wrong way on an interstate; the Standard-Gravure massacre in which a disgruntled pressman with an AK-47 slaughtered eight and wounded twelve; the Heath High School shooting where high school students in a morning prayer circle were shot by a freshman, killing three and injuring five others. These events and my involvement in them still affect me. I can still see the wounds and remember the victims' names, the details of their stories, and what it felt like to be there treating them. I still have waves of sadness sweep over me when I think of them, despite the fact that the most recent of these events occurred nearly twenty years ago. There are literally hundreds of other stories involving people for whom I have had the honor to care in my life as a doctor. These patients also had horrific injuries or diseases as well, but not so famously. Regardless, I carry them all.

There is a limbic system[4] response to all that we see and experience that isn't easily assuaged. It is the function of the amygdala to remember threats; it generalizes them and then applies that information to future events. Since the amygdala never forgets, humans are predisposed to anxiety and fear.[5] Fortunately, there is inhibitory input on the amygdala to help regulate its response through the prefrontal cortex.

Since the amygdala appears to be involved in the conscious experience of physical pain and emotional discomfort, our recognition of what is safe and what is dangerous runs through it. When you think about an impending fearful circumstance and are therefore, in

---

4   The limbic system lies between the cerebral cortex and the midbrain and is involved with memory, emotions, and learning. For our purposes, the amygdala and the hippocampus are this system's most important parts.

5   Louis Cozolino, *The Neuroscience of Psychotherapy: Healing the Social Brain* (New York: W. W. Norton, 2010), 254.

a sense, preparing for it, you have the capacity to inhibit the fear and/ or anxiety through the prefrontal cortex. The process can also work in the reverse: increased amygdala activation leads to less cortical activation. That could explain why it is hard to think when you are afraid. Extinction learning occurs when the memories housed in the amygdala are kept from activating the sympathetic nervous system through this higher inhibitory input.[6]

Stress can change the balance in the system. What has been extinguished can recur through the amygdala as a result of the suppression of the inhibitory input from the prefrontal cortex on the amygdala and the hippocampus, which provides context for these memories.[7] This provides a neural basis for the re-emergence of frightening experiences, even out of context, in the presence of prolonged or highly stressful situations. For instance, PTSD patients demonstrate an imbalance in the regulation of the limbic system from higher executive systems. Essentially, you can work and feel normal for a long time, but when subjected to prolonged stress or a highly stressful situation, past traumatic experiences can emerge through the amygdala. The emotion of that past experience is as real in the moment of recollection as when it originally occurred. The amplitude of reaction may be entirely disconnected from its trigger because your amygdala remembers the original danger. Behavioral and cognitive therapies are designed to increase the ability of the executive areas of the brain to inhibit the limbic system, specifically the amygdala.

Burnout is a distinct symptom of PTSD. However, childhood experiences in addition to the traumatic events of a physician's pro-

---

6   Ibid., 250–256.

7   W. Jacobs and L. Nadel, "Stress-Induced Recovery of Fears and Phobias," *Psychological Review* 92, no. 4, (October 1985), 512–531.

fessional life—which can predispose the development of PTSD—can increase the likelihood of a doctor experiencing symptoms of burnout because of the emotional dysregulation inherent in PTSD.

There is mounting evidence that burnout and PTSD may be linked. A study of firefighters found a relationship between work-related injuries, the Maslach Burnout Inventory's (a leading survey for measuring burnout) dimension of emotional exhaustion, and symptoms of PTSD.[8] The same study also found relationships between the Maslach Burnout Inventory's dimension of depersonalization and symptoms of PTSD.[9] A study in Israel found physicians who had symptoms of PTSD demonstrated more depression and anxiety and suffered greater burnout.[10] The study also found that the physicians were reluctant to seek treatment.[11]

BURNOUT BY THE NUMBERS

In spite of increasing awareness, physician burnout is reaching epidemic proportions—and the problem appears to be worsening. Burnout was first described in psychologist Herbert Freudenberger's 1974 article as the effect of work-related stress on job satisfaction.[12] It has since been characterized as a "state of mental and physical exhaustion related to work or caregiving activities."[13]

---

8   F. Katsavouni et al., "The Relationship between Burnout, PTSD symptoms and Injuries in Firefighters," *Occupational Medicine* 66, no. 1 (January 2016), 32–37.

9   Ibid.

10 Sharon Einav et al., "Differences in Psychological Effects in Hospital Doctors with and without Post-Traumatic Stress Disorder," *The British Journal of Psychiatry* 193, no. 2 (July 2008), 165–166.

11 Ibid.

12 Herbert Freudenberger, "Staff Burn-Out," *Journal of Social Issues* 30, no. 1 (January 1974).

13 Waguih William IsHak et al., "Burnout during Residency Training: A Literature Review," *Journal of Graduate Medical Education* 1, no. 2 (December 2009): 236–242, US National Library of Medicine, National Institutes of

Burnout, as defined by the social psychologist Christina Maslach, is a psychological syndrome that develops secondary to work-related stress and is characterized by emotional exhaustion, depersonalization, and a sense of reduced personal accomplishment,[14] something many physicians have felt. In fact, Medscape in 2015 released survey results on more than twenty thousand USA-based physicians across twenty-six specialties.[15] Overall, burnout was reported in nearly 46 percent of the survey participants, up from 39.8 percent in 2013.[16]

Between 2011 and 2014, the percentage of physicians reporting at least one burnout symptom increased from 45.5 to 54.4 percent.[17] Some specialties are hit harder. A 2008 survey of eight thousand surgeons found that nearly 40 percent of them met criteria for burnout.[18] The percentage of surgeons affected increased to 51 percent in the Medscape survey released in January 2016, which also reported that approximately 53 to 55 percent of emergency room physicians, critical care doctors, urologists, and pediatricians suffered from burnout.[19]

Health, accessed June 14, 2017, https://www.ncbi.nlm.nih.gov/pmc/articles/PMC2931238/#i1949-8357-1-2-236-Freudenberger1.

14   C. Maslach, S. E. Jackson, and M. P. Leiter, *Maslach Burnout Inventory Manual*, 3rd ed. (Palo Alto, CA: Consulting Psychologists Press, 1996).

15   Carol Peckham, "Physician Burnout: It Just Keeps Getting Worse," Medscape, January 26, 2015, accessed June 15, 2017, http://www.medscape.com/viewarticle/838437.

16   Ibid.

17   Tait D. Shanafelt et al., "Changes in Burnout and Satisfaction with Work-Life Balance in Physicians and the General US Working Population between 2011 and 2014," *Mayo Clinic Proceedings* 90 (2015), 1600–1613.

18   Tait D. Shanafelt et al., "Burnout and Career Satisfaction among American Surgeons," A*nnals of Surgery* 250, no. 3 (September 2009), 463–471, doi:10.1097/SLA.0b013e3181ac4dfd.

19   Carol Peckham, "Medscape Lifestyle Report 2016: Bias and Burnout," Medscape, January 13, 2016, accessed June 15, 2017, http://www.medscape.com/slideshow/lifestyle-2016-overview-6007335.

Specialists in fields such as dermatology, ophthalmology, and psychiatry had a lower percentage of respondents meeting burnout criteria in the 2016 survey. However, their rates of burnout, which were 40 to 43 percent, were higher than the average of 39.8 percent reported for all physicians in 2013.[20] Staggering statistics to be sure.

Residents are also adversely affected by burnout. General surgery residents have the highest burnout rates, followed by residents in radiology, surgical subspecialties, anesthesiology, and internal medicine. On at least one subscale of the Maslach Burnout Inventory—which looks at emotional exhaustion, depersonalization, and low sense of personal accomplishment—69 percent of residents in general surgery met the criterion for burnout.[21]

A 2006 study reported in *Academic Medicine* also found that burnout "appears common among U.S. medical students and may increase by year of schooling."[22] In addition to work-related stress, the study found that "personal life events also demonstrated a strong relationship to professional burnout."[23] Compared to college graduates of the same age, students in medical school reported higher rates of burnout in the study. An article in *The Atlantic Monthly* in 2014 reported that, specifically, these students suffer from emotional exhaustion, depersonalization, and a diminished sense of personal accomplishment at rates higher than their peers.[24] Personal matters

20 Ibid.
21 Jeffe Elmore et al., "National Survey of Burnout among US General Surgery Residents," *Journal of the American College of Surgeons* 223, no. 3 (September 2016): 440–451.
22 Liselotte Dyrbye et al., "Personal Life Events and Medical Student Burnout: A Multicenter Study," abstract, *Academic Medicine* 81, no. 4 (April 2006): 374–384, accessed June 15, 2017, http://journals.lww.com/academicmedicine/Abstract/2006/04000/Personal_Life_Events_and_Medical_Student_Burnout_.10.aspx.
23 Ibid.
24 Richard Gunderman, "For the Young Doctor about the Burn Out," *Atlantic Monthly* (February 21, 2014), accessed June 15, 2017, https://www.theatlantic.

and other factors related to curriculum were reported to be associated with the development of these symptoms in students.[25]

Physicians commit suicide more frequently than the general population—four hundred deaths per year—despite similar rates of depression and other associated mental illnesses. Reliable statistics do not yet exist, but many believe that the accurate number of physician suicides per year is much greater than the four hundred often cited. And rates of burnout are higher among female physicians, as are rates of suicide. For male physicians, the rate ratio for suicide is 1.4 versus the general population, and for female doctors it is 2.3.[26]

If the rates of depression and other mental illnesses are similar, why are the suicide rates higher? That's a disturbing question.

MY OWN BURNOUT

I was in danger of becoming a statistic. I made the decision to undergo intensive psychotherapy at an outpatient treatment facility only because I had suffered enough to realize, when confronted, that I needed help. When I arrived there, I was reassured to discover that there were a lot of other "normal-just-broken" guys like me. I felt a little like the fictional charlie-in-the-box of the renowned children's holiday movie *Rudolph the Red-Nosed Reindeer*. Like Charlie, who lived on the island of misfit toys, from the outside I looked and func-

com/health/archive/2014/02/for-the-young-doctor-about-to-burn-out/284005/.

25 Liselotte Dyrbye et al., "Burnout among U.S. Medical Students, Residents, and Early Career Physicians Relative to the General U.S. Population," *Academic Medicine* 89, no. 3 (March 2014), 443–451.

26 Tait D. Shanafelt et al., "Changes in Burnout and Satisfaction with Work-Life Balance in Physicians and the General US Working Population between 2011 and 2014," *Mayo Clinic Proceedings* 90, no. 12 (December 2015), 1600–1613, accessed June 15, 2017, http://www.mayoclinicproceedings.org/article/S0025-6196(15)00716-8/abstract.

tioned well. My issues were all beyond what could be seen, touched, and examined with the eye.

Still, psychotherapy was the last thing I—an accomplished surgeon—ever envisioned myself doing. But I was not alone. I met accomplished dentists, pharmacists, family physicians, surgeons, radiologists, anesthesiologists, and pathologists during my stay at this facility. All of them were professionals who needed help, and they were getting it.

Some refer to my journey as a recovery. I prefer to call it redemption, which *Merriam-Webster's Dictionary* defines as "serving to offset or compensate for a defect." That also encompasses the concept of a buy back, or an act of salvation. That's what I was trying to do: be redeemed from all that I had imposed on those who were closest to me, and get "me" back at the same time. Similar to the perimeter of the fallout from any sort of destructive or violent act, there is significant fallout around a physician, resident, or medical student who is suffering from burnout. Just as when a building implodes, the closer you are to the epicenter, the more you feel the effects. It is the same with burnout: The worse the burnout is, the more intensely it is felt by those closest to the individual suffering burnout, and the larger the sphere of destruction. It is impossible to suffer from emotional exhaustion, depersonalization, and dissatisfaction at work and not bring that suffering home, and the realization of how my actions had impacted my social sphere was an agonizing part of my healing journey.

Not surprisingly, I believe my fall affected my ability to function as a professional. I know my colleagues, patients, and the staff with whom I worked were, at times, adversely affected, even if it was just because of the manner in which I spoke or the attitude I projected. I felt most labile, in retrospect, when I had planned events a certain way and things did not go as I had expected or intended. An example might be those occasions when I would order a test or a scan to be done in a certain sequence, with the idea that I would have the information needed to make a clinical decision, and then the patient didn't show, or the insurance company denied the scan, or the technologist thought I wanted a different scan. My anger in these moments was palpable. I could, generally, avoid a classic rage—I wouldn't curse, or scream, or throw things—but I raged by allowing my erudite sarcasm to flow like lava. That allowed me to claim the high road, venting frustration on patients and staff. The same behavior happened at home, only when I was there I had a greater propensity to become sullen and not speak at all.

Evelyn, my wife, first vocalized that something was wrong with me a few months before we decided to go to counseling together. She suggested that I have a CT scan of my head done because she was concerned that I "might have a tumor or something." I laugh when I recall the discussion I had when I later visited my internist, who is also a good friend.

"I need a CT of the head," I told him.

"Why?" Jim asked.

"Evelyn says I need one."

"Okay, how do I code that?"

"I have the worst headache I have ever had," I stated flatly.

The CT was normal, of course.

I consider myself extremely fortunate to have never been sanctioned, disciplined, or brought before a committee or a board for disruptive behavior or any other incident. I also consider myself more fortunate—not more resilient, or better in any way—than many of my colleagues, whose bottoming out included DUIs, drug arrests, divorces, dismissal from hospital staffs, disciplining by medical boards, suicide, or many other more public displays of psychological unraveling. There I go, but for the grace of God.

Admittedly, revealing the truth of my journey is foreboding. I feel like a small boy who peers around a doorway into a room filled with adults: he fears entering the room and being seen, and yet he wants so much to do exactly that. In telling my story, I hope to help other members of the medical community remove their fear of emerging from the shadows. There is a freedom and vulnerability in the light, although its glare can be imposing.

In a significant sense, this book is about telling a story to get it out, removing the power of the fear inherent in being truly seen. When an attempt is made to silence fear, however, the truth that resides within gives rise to anxiety or distressed behavior. In the attempt to control events, we become distrustful, seeking our own will. Fear grants the opportunity to seek help, trust others, and gain wisdom through experience, thus developing discernment.[27] It is such a common human experience that it's almost unnecessary to admit that facing our fears is scary. After all, facing our fears is, in reality, facing our selves. In facing our limitations and desires, we are forced to take responsibility and prepare, which in turn assuages the fear.

Intimacy at its core is a reflection of the inherent human desire to be seen and known. I believe it is something we all want, even if that desire remains hidden or disguised. Admittedly, intimacy is something I want, but I refused to admit my desire for intimacy for years. While I wanted to be truly known or seen, I feared rejection and abandonment. That is, ultimately, what everyone fears. Unfortunately for me, the fear of rejection existed unacknowledged beneath

---

27   Chip Dodd, *The Voice of the Heart: A Call to Full Living*, 2nd ed. (Nashville: Sage Hill Resources, 2014), 91–98.

my consciousness. We come into this world believing that if we "show up" we will be loved. I had to ask myself what made me want to hide and not "show up," revealing the truth of my inner experience: toxic shame.

What is toxic shame? According to Chip Dodd, author and my lead counselor at the Center for Professional Excellence (CPE)—where my wife and I sought counseling, and where I ultimately received treatment—toxic shame begins in childhood: "A child needs to see the parents as good. However, if the parents do not meet the core needs of the child, to keep the parents good, the child will see himself as bad as a way of maintaining attachment. This is the beginning of toxic shame. A person cannot have toxic shame without first carrying the inner wound of abandonment."[28] That abandonment can take many forms: denying the emotions of the child, neglecting the needs of the child, denying the child's emotions, giving the child adult responsibilities, or expecting the child to perform beyond his or her abilities, among many others.[29] Unfortunately, too often we're told that if we show up, respect boundaries, and tell the truth about our inner experience, we will not be liked. So we learn to do things "right" instead of "truthfully."

True intimacy requires sincerity. The word *sincerity* is derived from words referring to wholeness and pouring out.[30] Relating sincerity to a "poured-out wholeness" aligns it with the idea of integrity, which includes the notion of not being divided. It reflects the sentiment poet and philosopher Mark Nepo once summarized:

---

28 Chip Dodd, "Who We Are Made to Be," notebook of personal correspondence with author, 1995.

29 Ibid.

30 Derived from the Latin sincerus. Etymology from Proto-Indo-European sin (cf. Latin simplex, and Sanskrit [sama: whole, together] and [grow] [cf. Sanskrit skir, from kir: pour out]), https://en.wiktionary.org/wiki/sincerus.

"Indeed, to be sincere is to strive for nothing to exist between inner and outer."[31]

Recently, while walking with my wife past a playground on a lovely afternoon, a child's cries from atop a slide rang out: "Katy, see me!" he cried. "Katy, see me! See me! Please see me!" His pleading was so full of desperation and urgency, yet so full of life, that my wife remarked how much she wanted to find Katy and ask her to comply with the boy's wishes.

I understood exactly how the young boy felt. I wanted someone to truly see me. I wanted to be known, to be rejoiced, and to be appreciated for who I was. I believe we all crave that sort of intimacy, and yet we also avoid it. I want to be known, yes, but I also want to remain opaque because it seems safer.

The desire for intimacy results in the type of invitation we all crave but almost uniformly avoid. I want you to know the real me, but I hide the real me, and then I punish you for not knowing me. You compliment me, and I reject that compliment because I know that you see only the mask I have created to hide my true self. I don that mask to hide my shame, my humanness, my neediness. I reject how I am made, not realizing that "this toxic shame is really a rejection of the image of God we all carry in our hearts."[32]

No human can see into me if I choose to remain opaque. We create false selves because we have learned to despise our true self. With intimacy comes vulnerability—and vulnerability is scary.

---

31 Mark Nepo, *Inside the Miracle: Enduring Suffering, Approaching Wholeness* (Louisville, CO: Sounds True, 2015), 164.

32 Chip Dodd, *The Voice of the Heart: A Call to Full Living*, 2nd ed. (Nashville: Sage Hill Resources, 2014), 101.

ART—THE LANGUAGE OF HEALING

As we all were, I was born with a natural ability to speak the language of the heart. In part because of what I suffered, and as a result because of the vows I made to myself to power through that suffering, that ability was suppressed. Prior to entering therapy, I didn't have a language to express what or how I felt. I had forgotten that speaking the language of the heart was important. At that point, my heart had no voice. Treatment gave back to me the words, the language, the voice that spoke the truth of my heart.

During treatment, I read the book *The Return of the Prodigal Son: A Story of Homecoming* by theologian and philosopher Henri Nouwen. The book is Nouwen's memoir, framed as a reflection on how his life was mirrored in a selection of paintings. The book spoke so powerfully to me that I realized there were several paintings that I had seen that spoke to me deeply about the two most dominant aspects of my own life—myself as a physician and as a person in recovery.

As I continued the process of healing following treatment, I began to encounter a surprising affinity for—and deep connection to—art. As someone who was prone to intellectualizing or rationalizing everything before treatment, an affinity for art would have been an intrusion into my psyche. Previously, I would have most certainly dismissed time spent on art as trivial, unimportant, and unnecessary. For instance, under that construct, reading historical treatises and biographies of great leaders and thinkers would have been an acceptable use of time, whereas art simply was not.

My interest in art was initially sparked by visiting the National Gallery of Art in London, while I was there to see my daughter during a semester when she was studying abroad. The affinity with art that I started to feel there grew into a passion. I became captivated, particularly with sixteenth- and seventeenth-century Renaissance art. Since I had routinely avoided art and art history classes in high school and college, I was all the more intrigued with, and curious about, what these paintings stirred in me, particularly when seeing them displayed in a museum. What I discovered is that the story I saw reflected in particular pieces granted me easier access to parts of my heart that had previously been difficult to reach. It felt as though I were dusting off an old shelf and finding hidden treasures.

So, art became an avenue to my feelings that centered on the story in the paintings, which resonated with a part of my own life story. Art gave me a symphonic canvas over which my heart was moved to sing. I began to get my heart's voice back.

RECONNECTING WITH BEAUTY

In my journey to connect art to my own life, I rediscovered beauty and how it can revive the human spirit. Beauty allowed me access to an emotional place that I didn't reach by looking at things from a purely scientific, medical standpoint.

Beauty and creativity touch me deeply because they subconsciously remind me of the divine spark inherent in the human heart. God breathed into man the breath of life.[33] The Latin word for breath is *spiritus*. It is the root from which we derive the word *spirituality*. We live by breathing. Thus, life is, in essence, a spiritual experience. It can be transformative, mystical, and emotional, but to be spiritual is to fully live. Noticing a daffodil in the spring, a toddler's giggle, the death of a friend or loved one—these are spiritual experiences, and moments like these exemplify what it means to be present. Experiencing and connecting with beauty in such a way as to stir emotions can

33 Genesis 2:7.

help to make me a fuller—if not better—human being, physician, citizen, friend, father, and husband.

The spiritual experience of a breath or breathing is a universal part of life that connects us all. In some ways, it is the underlying principle upon which many meditative practices are based. The Franciscan priest Richard Rohr wrote, "There is no Islamic, Christian, or Jewish way of breathing. There is no African, American, or Asian way of breathing. There is no rich or poor way of breathing."[34] Numerous perspectives affirm the proposition that a spiritual practice is the one indispensable thing that helps people overcome their problems.[35] Spirituality allows you to be present in the *now*, which is a hallmark of a mindfulness practice. That is the essence of keeping heart.

A part of me hopes that the telling of my tale might keep some from ever abandoning their heart in the first place, or from ever having to embark on a journey to find their heart again. Prevention is worth a pound of cure, after all. But I also recognize that all people, at some point in their life, are at risk of losing a piece of themselves. Although some never venture to regain what they lost, for those who attempt the trip, I hope my saga will serve as a guidepost of sorts to finding the way home.

This story is unique. It is, after all, my story. However, though the facts and details are different from those of your story, I hope that some aspect of my story rings true to you, causing you to pause and consider your own heart.

---

34   Richard Rohr, *The Naked Now* (New York: The Crossroad Publishing Company, 2009).

35   Dan Buettner, *The Blue Zones: Lessons for Living Longer from the People Who've Lived the Longest* (Washington, DC: National Geographic Society, 2008); James D. Lane, Jon E. Seskevich, and Carl F. Pieper, "Brief Meditation Training Can Improve Perceived Stress and Negative Mood," *Alternative Therapies in Health and Medicine* 13, no. 1 (2007), 38–44; *Alcoholics Anonymous,* 4th ed. (New York: Alcoholics Anonymous World Services, 2001), 83–86.

"ANYONE IN THERE?"

When Evelyn and I were ending a joint counseling session at the CPE, Stephen, our counselor, told us he thought he knew what the problem was. I didn't realize he had determined that I was the problem. He left the room for a minute, and when he returned he took us to the office of David "Chip" Dodd, the director of the CPE. Chip recommended that I come to the center for a three-day evaluation. He explained that the CPE was designed to minister to people in the "helping" professions who were successful at helping others but were nevertheless "impaired."

*I tuned out for a moment, focusing on the fact that I had just been labeled "impaired." Then Chip held his hand close to my face, waved it, snapped his fingers, and asked, "Anyone in there?" He spoke to a part of me that needed to be spoken to. "You can't give what you don't have, so we are going to help you get you back who you were made to **be**, so you can then go do what you were made to **do**: give to others," he said with a really big smile.*

"I don't know how I can get three days off," I said, "I have been elected to be the Kentucky Medical Association president in September." Chip broke in, "You will be a better husband, better father, better doctor, and a better KMA president if you come in."

I decided to do it, and Evelyn was incredibly supportive. The idea of "getting me back so I could do what I was made to do" was irresistible to me—I had longed for that, and Chip touched on it in a matter of minutes. I was willing to risk discomfort and did the impossible: I rearranged my schedule to get three days off.

FIND YOUR
HEART

As you examine your own situation, remember these points:

- Burnout can be a slow leak punctuated by multiple traumatic episodes. It *does not* have to be associated with drug or alcohol abuse, disruptive behavior, or a history of mental illness.

- We have a tendency to develop defenses to protect our hearts. This happens because we have been wounded. However, a guarded heart does not allow for the full expression of emotions. This is a denial of our humanness.

- Connecting with beauty through art or other activities can facilitate the expression of emotions that have been difficult to access previously.

- Spirituality/mindfulness is essential to developing nonjudgmental awareness

Consider these exercises to help you on your own healing journey:

- Write a half-page paragraph for each of the five most painful events of your life.

- Did you make any promises or vows to yourself as a result of each of these experiences? If so, what were these vows? Can you see how they may have been temporarily beneficial but have become harmful to your heart?

- Sometimes we avoid activities that bring us the greatest joy and connect us in a meaningful way to the person we truly are. We avoid these endeavors because they don't help the monthly budget, they don't make sense, they're silly, no one does them, we don't have time for them, and even because they can be painful or uncomfortable despite the joy they bring. Can you think of some activities you have avoided or neglected participating in despite the joy they bring you? Write them down and the reasons you give your self for not doing them.

TWO

BEFORE THE HIGH PRIEST: THE STORY OF THE ACCUSED AND HIS ACCUSER

When you blame and criticize others, you are avoiding some truth about yourself.

—Deepak Chopra

Many poets are not poets for the same reason that many religious men are not saints: they never succeed in being themselves.

—Thomas Merton

I heard the crack as the ball struck the bat, and I could immediately discern that the ball was mine. The pop-up was coming directly to me. I was standing just a few steps off third base, and I called out to all of the other infielders, "I got it, I got it." At that moment, I heard a little voice whisper, "If you drop this ball, Dad will kill you." Those fly balls that make you stand there and wait for them to come down were always the most difficult for me—it gives you too much time to think. I concentrated a little harder, centered myself under the ball, and kept an eye on it just as my father had taught me. As it nestled into the webbing of my glove, I grasped it firmly, quickly covering the ball with my right hand just to make sure it didn't sneak out.

I blushed to myself as I thought about that surprising little voice whispering to me as the ball was still soaring upward. I was forty-two years old at the time, and playing on my ear, nose, and throat (ENT) office's softball team. My father was in the stands; he had come to watch us play. There was obviously still a huge part of me that wanted to please him, or perform for him, even then.

My father—also known as Sweet William, Pedro, Lego, Bill, Billy, Andy, and Andrew—had coached me in baseball until high school. He threw batting practice for hours on end, sometimes pitching to my whole team on his days off. He was a sergeant in the Kentucky State Police, which is the same rank he held when he was in the army. He had served in between the Korean War and the Vietnam conflict. The Cuban Missile Crisis was as close as he came to war, unless you consider being raised by an alcoholic a type of war. His father, my grandfather, was rarely at home in Lockport, Kentucky. In those days, during the Great Depression, Lockport was a rough river town in Henry County, near a lock on the Kentucky River. When my grandfather was home, more often than not he was drunk and beating his sons—my dad and his older brother—or my grandmother. Occasionally, he beat all three at the same time.

When I think about my own childhood in retrospect, whether intentional or not, the messages I received from my parents led me to believe their acceptance of me was conditional and based on performance. That's what came to me in that baseball game during adulthood. As I stood there, waiting for that infield pop-up, I recognized for the first time that my inner voice was not my own; it was my father's. As thought leader Peggy O'Mara said, "The way we talk to our children becomes their inner voice." The idea that I am implanting an inner voice in my own children scares me to death.

Family of origin is important in psychodynamics; it is a significant factor in the development of resilience. Your background may be different than mine, but your family experiences are an underlying factor in your later journey in life. They may help determine how—or not—you cope with burnout. The human need to *be* and the need to *matter* are more important that the need for food, clothing, and shelter. You learn from your family how to "behave." By that I do *not* mean "doing as you are told," I mean "to have being." What you learn is how to be "you." The need for relationships is so powerful that children sometimes lose their identities, their true selves, just to have it. Sometimes, they even lose their lives because of the need for relationships.[36]

In my own childhood, I began to equate punishment with rejection, which I wanted to avoid at all costs. I really wanted to be "good." As a result, I lost contact with my own feelings, desires, longings, and needs. I lost me, and didn't know it. But I had to lose me to please my parents, to be "good." Theologian Thomas Merton wrote:

> For you sanctity consists in being your self ... For me to be a saint means to be myself. Therefore the problem of sanctity and salvation is in fact the problem of finding out who I am and of discovering my true self.
>
> Trees and animals have no problem. God makes them what they are without consulting them, and they are perfectly satisfied.

---

36 Chip Dodd, private communication.

With us it is different. God leaves us free to be whatever we like. We can be ourselves or not, as we please. We are at liberty to be real, or to be unreal. We may be true or false, the choice is ours. We may wear now one mask and now another, and never, if we so desire, appear with our own true face. But we cannot make these choices with impunity.[37]

During therapy I came to a deeper understanding of the concept of inner voice, and found to my relief that I am not my inner voice; I am not the critic. My true self lies much deeper within me than that. According to Zen masters, the "face you had before you were born" is what is revealed when the inner thoughts are quieted. "Your True Self is who you objectively are, from the beginning in the mind and heart of God."[38] My true self, or the real me, is not the inner voice that is so often accusatory. That characteristic alone should help discern who is really responsible for that voice. It is the accuser.[39]

THE PAINTING

Gerrit van Honthorst, a Dutch Golden Age artist, painted *Christ before the High Priest* in the early part of the seventeenth century. Honthorst was skilled at chiaroscuro, a technique that features dramatic contrasts between light and dark areas on the canvas. It was a style influenced by

---

37 Thomas Merton, *New Seeds of Contemplation* (New York: New Directions Publishing, 1961), 31–32.

38 Richard Rohr, *Falling Upward: A Spirituality for the Two Halves of Life* (San Francisco: Jossey-Bass, 2011), 86.

39 This is Satan. The Hebrew noun "Satan" usually signifies "adversary." The verb form also means "to accuse." The name Satan is transliterated "diábolos" many times in the New Testament to conform with the LXX (Septuagint translators). They appeared to have chosen this term, which we translate into English as 'devil,' because its root meaning is "to accuse." (Geoffery Bromiley, *International Standard Bible Encyclopedia* 4 (1979), 342.)

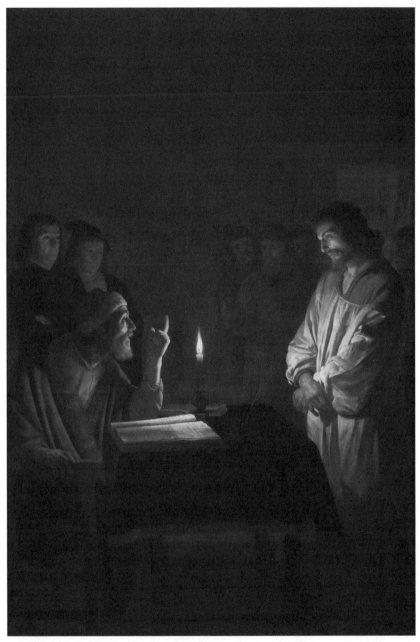

Christ before the High Priest, Gerrit van Honthorst

the Italian artist Michelangelo Merisi da Caravaggio, and one which probably gained Honthorst some degree of fame while in Rome.

Following his death, Honthorst was often referred to as *Gherardo delle notti*, or Gerard of the night, for his depiction of artificially lit scenes such as the one in this masterpiece, which is illuminated by a single candle. The painting shows the night of Christ's trial. It is the story of the accused and his accuser. Conceptually, it's a metonymy for everything that accuses, including the inner voice.

When I saw this painting, it was Jesus's serenity that first drew my attention. His robe jumps off the canvas with its light color. The right hand of Caiphas is near the center of the painting and is illuminated strongly by the light of the candle, also near the center of the scene. The emotions stirred within me by this painting are conflicted and strong, as is the biblical passage that the masterpiece portrays, Matthew 26:57:

> And those who had laid hold of Jesus led Him away to Caiaphas, the high priest, where the scribes and the elders were assembled. But Peter followed Him at a distance to the high priest's courtyard. And he went in and sat with the servants to see the end.
>
> Now the chief priests, the elders, and all the council sought false testimony against Jesus to put Him to death, but found none. Even though many false witnesses came forward, they found none. But at last two false witnesses came forward and said, "This fellow said, 'I am able to destroy the temple of God and to build it in three days.'"
>
> And the high priest arose and said to Him, "Do You answer nothing? What is it these men testify against You?" But Jesus kept silent. And the high priest answered and said to Him, "I put You under oath by the living God: Tell us if You are the Christ, the Son of God!"

Jesus said to him, "It is as you said. Nevertheless, I say to you, hereafter you will see the Son of Man sitting at the right hand of the Power, and coming on the clouds of heaven."

Then the high priest tore his clothes, saying, "He has spoken blasphemy! What further need do we have of witnesses? Look, now you have heard His blasphemy! What do you think?"

They answered and said, "He is deserving of death."[40]

The perfunctory nature of the proceedings is laid bare in the text through phrases such as "sought false testimony" and "false witnesses came forward." The implication in the text is that people may indeed find what they seek, perhaps giving rise to the well-known saying, "Be careful what you wish for."

If you find it difficult to admit what you seek, as I do, it is nevertheless a good thing to be curious about your motivations. It not only can help you gain a more realistic appraisal of yourself, but it can help you know others better as well. As the Swiss psychiatrist and psychoanalyst Carl Jung said, "Knowing your own darkness is the best method for dealing with the darknesses of other people."

There is more than meets the eye in the play between lightness and darkness in the painting. The dramatic illumination of the room via the single candle brilliantly serves multiple purposes, including allowing the witnesses or liars to lurk appropriately in the darkness, or the shadows, at the margins of the action depicted in the center of the composition.

The two individuals who at last come forward in the text are undoubtedly the figures behind the high priest in the painting. They

---

40   Matthew 26:57–66 (New King James Version).

are "in darkness" but unaware of their own darkness. It is apparent that they have not had a transformative experience that can only be accessed through the kind of direct healing resulting from an active inner world.[41] When I admit my own reticence to engage in that inner world, it causes sadness, guilt, fear, and hurt to wash over me.

The candle also allows a somewhat reddish hue to imbue the painting, which intensifies as the eye drifts from the center. While the two figures are on the side of the High Priest Caiaphas, both physically and metaphorically, the primary accuser is undoubtedly Caiaphas, who is seated and appears to be speaking. His eyebrows are raised and his forehead is wrinkled. His hand, almost glowing from the intensity of the candle, is raised above a book, a pointing finger seemingly emphasizing his words. That book is the Law of God, most assuredly the Torah. It is no coincidence that the brightest parts of the painting are the book, the candlelight itself, and the robe of our Lord. The very words He wrote are used to accuse Him.

It's sad that truth and uprightness are often used by those in positions of power to accuse others whom they can accuse only as a result of their position, as though people's personal power can hide their darkness from them and yet allow them to feel justified when they project it onto others. How self-deluded Caiaphas was to raise his illuminated finger over the Law of God as he accused the sinless lamb, the Light of the World, of violating the very words He had penned. It saddens me to recognize how power can hide my darkness from me. And when I project that darkness onto others, as Caiaphas did, I can feel justified in making the accusation. "You can forgive

---

41   Robert Moore and Doug Gillette, *King, Warrior, Magician Lover: Rediscovering the Archetypes of the Mature Masculine* (New York; Harper Collins, 1990), 3.

the outer world only if and when you have first forgiven your own inner world."[42]

THE VOICES THAT ACCUSE

An Old Testament prophet wrote, "Then he showed me Joshua the high priest standing before the angel of the Lord, and Satan standing at his right side to accuse him."[43] The passage states that it is Satan's purpose to accuse. If Satan is willing to accuse Jesus, then a high priest is certainly not immune to such an act. Satan certainly slandered Job, and he certainly attacks our hearts.

Yet, it can sometimes seem as if there are enough voices to fill a chorus in joining Satan as he sings his accusations against you. Those voices can take the tone, rhythm, and cadence of parents, siblings, other family and friends, mentors, and colleagues. For physicians, they can take the form of patients and other associates. They can even sound like the physician's own voice.

At times, all of these voices seem to have accused me. But as spiritual teacher Eckhart Tolle says, "What a liberation to realize that the 'voice in my head' is not who I am. Who am I then? The one who sees that." There is an inner observer who recognizes the voice of accusation. That is me. Meditation practices, centering, and contemplative prayer can help to achieve a sense of objectless awareness or nondual consciousness, which allows the ego to dissipate. Since everyone has inner critics, then we are all, in essence, in the same

---

42 Richard Rohr, *Immortal Diamond: The Search for Our True Self* (San Francisco: Jossey-Bass, 2013), 48.

43 Zechariah 3:1.

boat. But there is data to suggest that people who have a more active critical inner voice are more subject to depression.[44]

When people's words are used against them, as is often the case when accused, it is difficult not to feel anger. How often do they honestly deserve such accusations? How do they respond when falsely accused? What about those times when they are justifiably accused? Jesus remained perfectly calm, completely aware of who He was. So what is it that makes the rest of us bristle, become defensive and indignant, and seek to question, vindicate, justify, or explain?

These questions arose in me a few years back, following an incident that happened after I received a phone call from a colleague who was a cardiovascular surgeon. He said he had a favor to ask. He was developing a wildflower garden on the land next to his house and had hired out some of the heavier landscaping to a man with whom he had become relatively good friends. His friend's teenage son had been suffering from an ear infection, which my colleague had tried to treat, unsuccessfully. I agreed to give the boy an ENT evaluation, working him into an already overbooked and busy schedule. Plus, at my friend's request, I did not charge for my services since the family did not have insurance. There was, and still remains, a fairly sizeable uninsured population in this area of Kentucky, and without an academic university hospital nearby, it is not uncommon for physicians to provide care regardless of the patient's inability to pay.

When the teen and his father came to see me, they were very personable and appreciative, especially since the boy was in considerable pain. I was able to diagnose his problem relatively quickly and took the steps I thought necessary to resolve the infection. I gave him

---

44 Lisa Firestone, "The Critical Inner Voice That Causes Depression," *Psychology Today* (blog), September 28, 2010, accessed September 9, 2017, https://www.psychologytoday.com/blog/compassion-matters/201009/the-critical-inner-voice-causes-depression.

sample antibiotics and some eardrops so they would not have to pay for any medication.

I recommended that they come back for a follow-up visit a week later. The teen informed his dad that he wouldn't be available then. When I asked why, his dad replied, "He has been looking forward to this trip to Honduras for a long time. He leaves in a couple of days and won't be back in time."

Immediately, I thought, *Wait a minute. Here I am providing free care to someone who can afford to go on vacation to someplace I've never even been. He'll be climbing the Mayan ruins at Copan and playing on the beaches of Roatán, and I'll be stuck here in this office.*

Now, I am not known for being a reserved person. In fact, I tend to be pretty outspoken. But, at that moment, I managed to contain my dismay—and welling-up disdain—and, instead, suggested that they return right before he was to leave. "That way I will have an opportunity to change things around a bit if you haven't quite resolved this infection," I said. They both thanked me profusely and left, and I returned to helping patients and completely forgot about the young man and his father.

A couple of days later, a nurse stopped me in the hall and informed me that she had seen the young man and his father at church. "They were singing your praises," the nurse said. "His ear feels completely better. And he is so excited about going on that mission trip to Honduras. The whole church is paying for all the youth to go on it. They said you were even going to see him again before he left to make sure he was well. They could not say enough good things about you." I thanked the nurse for sharing the good news with me, and I immediately felt extremely fortunate that, for once in my life, I had kept my thoughts to myself.

In my mind, I had accused and judged both the father and the young man. I judged them out of a sense of envy, from a position of power and privilege—in part, the same factors that caused Caiaphas to judge and accuse Jesus. What is worse?

BEING ACCUSED

As I said earlier, I've also been on the other side of the accusations, where Jesus stood. The difference is I have rarely been accused innocently. To be honest, I have often done things as bad or worse than that of which I have been accused.[45] The Lord was different.

As an intern, I was on call in general surgery every other night for six months. One of the attending physicians at the hospital where I interned had trained with Chester McVay, MD, who developed a classic procedure to repair inguinal hernias. The attending physician, Dr. Johnson, was a skilled anatomist as well as an academic surgeon.

I felt lucky because I had obtained a copy of McVay's two-volume anatomy text. My assignment to scrub with Dr. Johnson was five days away. I was to be on call the night before the procedure, but, up to that point, I read everything I could get my hands on about the procedure, including the anatomy, complications, and recovery. I also read up on Dr. McVay and his record of service in World War II. Turned out it was a really smart move to read everything beforehand, because the trauma team I was on got hammered the day and night before the procedure. I did not see my call room all night.

When I turned over the beeper to the intern on the call team following me, I had just enough time to look at the patient's chart, pre-op, and get the patient in position before Dr. Johnson's arrival. I was really excited to be learning from a man who had trained with

---

45 Romans 3:23.

a giant in the field, but I was also eager to demonstrate my study and mastery of the material required to perform the operation. Who knew? I might even get to throw a stitch or two. Admittedly, I was exhausted, but I was also pumped by a rush of adrenaline.

I scrubbed and went in to wait for Dr. Johnson, who was known to be a no-nonsense guy. When he came in, I said good morning and introduced myself. He looked me up and down. He turned away from me to face the nurse who was helping him gown and asked me, without turning to face me, "Did you read about hernias last night?"

Hesitantly, I said, "No, but I—"

"You nothing!" he screamed, whipping around as he tied his gown. "And I mean 'you nothing!' You are nothing and you will do nothing today. Get out of my operating room and do not *ever* step foot in it again unprepared."

There was no debating, no arguing. It was a waste of breath. I left angry. I was angry at him for being so arrogant, unreasonable, and demanding. I was angry at myself for not stealing away the night before to read for five or ten minutes. I was angry that I had told the truth; he would have never known—but I would have.

As a medical professional in training, you stand accused. Everything is reviewed and critiqued. Physicians spend their lives wanting to help others, but, as humans, they sometimes make mistakes. In today's world, that means litigation and accusations of intent. In such an environment, students often become their own harshest critic, but there are plenty of people in the chorus, which can lead to physicians being more critical of others as well as themselves.

Part of the wounding from that incident was that it touched me in a very tender place—my toxic shame. He merely reinforced what I already thought about myself.

PHYSICIAN, LOVE THYSELF

A key to healing is to love others. And the key to loving others is to love yourself first; you can only be as kind to others as you are to yourself. Perhaps that is the meaning of loving your neighbor as yourself.[46] Healthy shame merely tells us we need help. It tells me, "I don't know everything, and neither do you. Let's work together."

People experience toxic shame when they feel inherently deficient and unlovable. It is possible for toxic shame to become a part of one's core identity as a result of how they were raised by their parents. Adults who were shamed when growing up carry their wounds into their roles as mothers and fathers, and they pass the hurt on. Children learn to perform in order to be accepted, externalizing their worth. Closing the heart protects it against the feeling of worthlessness, of suffering, but it takes us away from our feelings, away from our self.

Another word for suffering, in Greek, is passion.[47] In one sense, passion is a kind of anger. In the painting, Christ realizes that his purpose is not going to be served by any significant response to the accusations. He does not display anger, the way we usually think of it, though He does have passion. He has a higher purpose than anyone in the room realizes, and that enables him to suffer while keeping his ultimate purpose in focus. Anger conveys what matters to us. Aside from demonstrating passion, anger reflects what we care about and provides the elan to be truly present.[48] Jesus is completely in possession of himself and, in suffering, serves the world.

Much of life is about learning how to deal with loss, about how to suffer well. Suffering well can be thought of as "living life on life's

---

46   Leviticus 19:17.

47   πάθο (pathos).

48   Chip Dodd, *The Voice of the Heart: A Call to Full Living*, 2nd ed. (Nashville: Sage Hill Resources, 2014), 79–82.

terms," a phrase often heard in twelve-step meetings. Alcoholics Anonymous (AA) meetings are generally thought to be for alcoholics and addicts. The surprising thing I discovered while attending those meetings during my treatment was how many people medicate with something besides alcohol: drugs, the facade of control, power, money, sex, superficial religion. The list is endless. People medicate to numb themselves to the reality they don't like, the feelings they don't want to feel. We want to go away, but there is no such place as "away" when it comes to emotions.

As a physician, can you suffer well? When you walk into a room where a patient who is dying of cancer takes his frustration and anger out on you, can you recognize that patient is not angry at you but, rather, at his situation? Can you put yourself in the shoes of such patients and realize that you'd be angry too? What I'm talking about is, of course, empathy, which is different than feeling sorry for patients. Feeling sorry for them is sympathy. Author and scholar Brené Brown calls being sympathetic similar to saying, "I don't understand your world, but from this view things look pretty bad."[49] Sympathy preserves separation, and can even heighten feelings of shame in the one to whom the sympathy is given. How can you suffer in service to others without depleting your reservoir of emotional energy? Empathic concern or compassion connects us as humans, bridges experiences at a heart level, and says, "I understand how that feels." Empathy is having the ability to effectively communicate that understanding, and then having a desire to help. It is like "feeling for" with action. Compassion, or empathy, requires having a handle on your own emotional world. I need to "have me" to be able to "give

---

49   Brené Brown, *I Thought It Was Just Me, (But It Isn't)* (New York: Penguin Random House, 2007), 51.

me." This is what Chip promised the day I first met him: to help me get back "me."

I believe this reveals an important paradox. I must lose or discard my false self or ego to lay bare my true self. I must lose myself to find myself.[50] I have to have myself to understand "how that feels." I cannot truthfully have compassion or empathic concern without having "me." Connecting with a patient empathically, then, moves me to help.[51]

SEEING BEAUTY IN OTHERS

When I came to the CPE, I stood accused. I accused myself for failing as a human being, for not being able to cope, for breaking down or burning out, though I had no idea at the time what my problems were. I even felt ashamed for not being able to suffer in a way that kept anyone from noticing. I felt I should have been stronger or better.

I was afraid, abjectly terrified, but that was all I was feeling. And yet it was pent-up fear, safely contained, controlled inside me. In my counselor's room, I stoically sat on the couch observably unperturbed by the proceedings. Just how I liked it.

*"Tell me about a beautiful thing you have seen or witnessed," my counselor said. Something about his question irritated me. I wanted to reach up and slap the smug look off his face.[52] I paused for a rather long time. **Perhaps the best response is just whatever pops into my head**, I thought. Risky, but I was out of options because I didn't really know what he wanted.*

---

50   Matthew 10:39.

51   This empathic concern, which results in altruistic behavior, activates reward centers in the brain. Thus, empathy can become a source of resilience helping to prevent burnout, whereas empathic distress will contribute to burnout. The difference between empathic concern and empathic distress is that, in empathic distress, we feel with the other person but do not recognize that the feelings are arising in the other person. Empathic concern recognizes that the feelings are originating from the other.

52   The feeling demonstrated here is anger.

At first, I told him about watching the sunrise with my family on a trip to the Grand Canyon. "It was pretty incredible," I told him.

"I'll bet it was," he replied. "Now tell me about something beautiful that touched you in a more intimate way, something more recent."

I was ready to scream. For someone who was used to always having all the answers, it was frustrating to lack the words, but even more so to not know the "right answer."

I thought about it for a moment and then began. "A few weeks ago, I was watching my oldest son play basketball at an away game. In the first few minutes of the game, my son's team was running its offense and he opened up for a three-point shot. He missed everything: the rim, the net, and the backboard. Predictably, a chant arose around the gym, 'air ball, air ball, air ball.' Another opportunity came up during their next offensive possession. My son's team ran the same play and he came open just as he had before. That time, he drained the shot. It was beautiful."

"What did you find beautiful about that?" my counselor asked.

"His courage. His heart in that was breathtaking. To do that in that kind of hostile environment was incredible. He amazed me." I teared up, and it honestly surprised me a little that so much emotion was in that experience for me.

"So, I do not believe you are a narcissist," my counselor calmly reported. I asked him why. "What you thought was beautiful, what touched you, wasn't about you and you didn't make it about you." I was not aware that narcissism was a diagnosis under consideration. I was glad he didn't think I was a narcissist, but honestly angry that it had entered his mind to check.

At that moment, a little part of me loosened my grip on the handlebars, just a bit. I was a little less terrified, maybe even a little more trusting. That was the first time I felt life might actually get better. A little gladness crept into my anger. I sensed hope.

FIND YOUR
HEART

- Journal what it would mean for you to be able to be yourself. What truth about yourself might you be avoiding?

- Do you have a tendency to intellectualize events to avoid discomfort? What is the price you pay for emotional detachment?

- Make a list of twenty-five things you are angry about. What do these things reveal about you?

- Would you like your life to be different? If so, how?

- The ability of Jesus to be fully present and in possession of himself in the face of hostile accusations is remarkable. What are the things in His life that you can emulate and that would assist you in developing this type of presence in the face of hostility?

- The words "You can forgive the outer world only if and when you have first forgiven your own inner world" are from page 32. How does this quotation speak to you and your ability to exhibit compassion?

- The pervasive nature of burnout and the factors that lead to it in the medical profession argue for mitigation strategies that incorporate individual and organizational approaches. As an individual, consider meditation, spirituality, and compassion training. Resources are listed in the bibliography at the end of the book.

THREE

CHRIST HEALING THE PARALYTIC: A SICK MAN AND HIS HEALER

First there is the fall and then there is the recovery
from the fall. But both are the mercy of God.

—Julian of Norwich

I first saw *Christ Healing the Paralytic at the Pool of Bethesda* by Bartolomé Esteban Murillo at the National Gallery of Art in London while on vacation with my family in the spring of 2010. This masterpiece represents the act of visiting the sick. Hospitals, of course, care for the infirm. The story this painting tells, and the manner of the telling, along with the parallels to my own life, were incredibly compelling. Just as the lame man lamented for "decades" that he had no one to help him enter the Pool of Bethesda, it was later revealed to me that healing wouldn't occur until I admitted I needed help. My heart's first experience of this painting was one of deep sadness. I was sad because my life had become unmanageable. The depth of that sadness spoke to me about how much I valued what I had lost.[53]

---

53   I had lost access to my feelings, my heart, authentic living. Essentially, I had lost me.

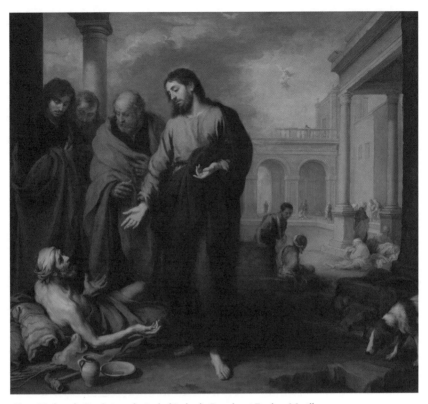

Christ Healing the Paralytic at the Pool of Bethesda, Bartolomé Esteban Murillo

The painting is large—seven feet nine inches by eight feet nine inches—and the figures are nearly life size. Displayed alone on a wall and hung approximately three feet off the floor, the presentation causes its subjects to loom larger than life. It is stunning.

Murillo was commissioned by the brotherhood of the Hospital de la Caridad (charity hospital) in Seville, Spain, to paint six large pieces for the church, representing six of the seven corporal acts of charity or mercy.[54] The seventh act is represented by a stunning baroque altarpiece. Two of the paintings still remain in the church.

---

54 The seven corporal acts of mercy are visiting the sick, redeeming the captive, sheltering pilgrims, clothing the naked, feeding the hungry, giving drink to the thirsty, and burying the dead.

The other four, including *Christ Healing the Paralytic at the Pool of Bethesda*, are now in various museums.

Murillo's masterpiece portrays the passage from John 5:1–15, in which Jesus heals a man afflicted with astheneia:

> After this there was a feast of the Jews, and Jesus went up to Jerusalem. Now there is in Jerusalem by the Sheep Gate a pool, which is called in Hebrew, Bethesda, [a] having five porches. In these lay a great multitude of sick people, blind, lame, paralyzed, waiting for the moving of the water. For an angel went down at a certain time into the pool and stirred up the water; then whoever stepped in first, after the stirring of the water, was made well of whatever disease he had. [b] Now a certain man was there who had an infirmity thirty-eight years. When Jesus saw him lying there, and knew that he already had been in that condition a long time, He said to him, "Do you want to be made well?"
>
> The sick man answered Him, "Sir, I have no man to put me into the pool when the water is stirred up; but while I am coming, another steps down before me."
>
> Jesus said to him, "Rise, take up your bed and walk." And immediately the man was made well, took up his bed, and walked.
>
> And that day was the Sabbath. The Jews therefore said to him who was cured, "It is the Sabbath; it is not lawful for you to carry your bed." He answered them, "He who made me well said to me, 'Take up your bed and walk.'"

Then they asked him, "Who is the Man who said to you, 'Take up your bed and walk?'" But the one who was healed did not know who it was, for Jesus had withdrawn, a multitude being in that place.

Afterward Jesus found him in the temple, and said to him, "See, you have been made well. Sin no more, lest a worse thing come upon you." The man departed and told the Jews that it was Jesus who had made him well.[55]

In Greek, *astheneia* can be translated as "weakness" or "disease," and does not necessarily imply a paralytic, as indicated in the painting's English title. *Bethesda* is derived from the Hebrew for "house of mercy." There is archeological evidence that this pool had originally been associated with a pagan Asclepion cult, whose symbol was a snake around a staff. Greek culture had extended its Hellenistic influences throughout the Mediterranean from the time of Alexander the Great.

How fitting that our Lord went to a pagan site whose inspiration was undoubtedly related to the brazen serpent Moses had lifted up in the wilderness,[56] whose likeness He would share.[57] Jesus goes there looking for a hopeless, debilitated brother whose own doings had, in all likelihood, placed him there by the pool.[58]

HOPE AND HOPELESSNESS

Whatever the malady the man was actually suffering from, it was of longstanding duration (some thirty-eight years). His incapacitation

---

55 John 5:1–15.
56 Numbers 21:6–9.
57 John 3:14.
58 John 5:14.

was evident from his hopelessness, which he freely admitted. Yet he hoped beyond hope. After all, he continued coming to the pool even though he expressed his condition in language that is reflective of his despair.[59] What choice did he have?

I have felt the same way. The only difference between myself and the paralytic was that he was far more self-aware. The paralytic knew he had astheneia. I did not recognize that I was weak and diseased.

Hurt as well as sadness welled up in me as I stood before the painting and considered the invalid's state of affliction. His position in the piece, below our Lord and the apostles, conveys his status in society as a result of his infirmity. His body language evinces his resignation, his sense of feeling trapped. Disease—or "dis-ease," with respect to his body and the apparent social injustice of his plight—left him bereft of awareness as to his inherent personal value. He dared not wish for more.

I have had that same "no-way-out" feeling, rising every day to perform the same rituals while hoping and praying that something would change. *Merriam-Webster's Dictionary* defines hopelessness as a) having no expectation of good or success, despairing; b) not susceptible to remedy or cure; c) incapable of redemption or improvement. I have always been taught that there is nothing beyond redemption, and yet have felt as though I were beyond the reach of redemption many times. I have felt a deep sense of hopelessness, as if the world were imploding. It is a suffocating feeling.

---

59 While it is true that some manuscripts omit the end of John 5:3 and all of verse 4, it is also true that the event (and the man's words in John 5:7) would make little sense if these words were eliminated. Why would anybody, especially a man sick for so many years, remain in one place if nothing special were occurring? You would think that after thirty-eight years of nothing happening to *anybody,* the man would go elsewhere and stop hoping! It seems wisest for us to accept the fact that something extraordinary kept all these people with disabilities at this pool, hoping for a cure (Warren Wiersbe BE Bible Study Series).

As a physician, it is easy to become frustrated[60] when dealing with disease. The odds are stacked against us. We fight an inevitably losing battle. When I was a young practitioner, I treated an elderly diabetic with a foot ulcer that I soaked and wrapped nearly every day for what seemed like an eternity. I vividly recall entering the patient's room one day. The oak floors creaked as I reluctantly inched my way toward her, step by step. As I drew closer, I sensed there was something unusual this particular afternoon.

Wrapped in a crocheted shawl, she was slowly rocking. Her long, speckled, black hair was curled in a tight weave, like a fine Tabriz, and looped into a bun. She shivered and greeted me lovingly, as she always did. I knelt and gently unfurled the gauze that had been carefully wrapped around her extended right foot. I was suddenly punched in the nose by a smell I could only imagine must have been comparable to a thousand rotting corpses. The uncharacteristic odor quickly permeated the room. I did not know then what it heralded but learned quickly that it meant an amputation. The patient died postoperatively, following a heart attack.

The patient was my great-grandmother, and even though I was only nine years old at the time, I distinctly recall the feeling of failure. We could have done better, done something different, sooner, faster, smarter. The truth is there was nothing more that could have been done, but I felt responsible anyway. Some of that responsibility I certainly assumed because I accompanied my mother on these frequent visits to care for my great-grandmother, and Mom felt responsible for the failure.

Even at that young age I knew I wanted to be a doctor. In spite of all that's occurred—the impact on my own mental and spiritual

---

60 While in treatment, I once remarked that I was not angry, just frustrated. Frustration, I was told, was Christianized anger.

health, spending my twenties in a library or an operating room—I would do it all over again. There are many other things about that journey that I would change were it possible, but I have always felt I was born to this calling. It was a desire placed within me that I had no choice but to follow, or I would suffer the consequences of refusal. You see, either way, there is suffering. There is a cost both to following desire and refusing it. There is no avoidance of suffering.

SETTING BOUNDARIES

Accepting responsibility—and guilt—for others' failures is a trait of many practitioners. How do you stop a smoker from smoking when he needs radiation therapy for a small vocal cord cancer? How do you get a diabetic with an Hgb A1C of 8.2 to eat a healthier diet? How do you convince motorcyclists to wear helmets? How do physicians persuade legislators that the innocent are protected when smoking in public places is restricted? How do we reach teenagers and make them aware of the hazards of drinking and driving, drinking and fighting, or drinking and swimming, boating, riding, walking, living? I have seen too much death and disability in the emergency department, and I have wept at my inability to change others' behaviors. Ironically, the things for which I need to take responsibility are often, if not always, the very things for which I desperately tried to avoid taking responsibility.

In the face of suffering for caring too much, the only alternative seems to be becoming calloused to the suffering of others, to not be a caring practitioner.[61] Patients commonly hope for a cure but often don't take an active role in their own health or healing. For the

---

61   In part, I believe we physicians battle death, an entity described in scripture as "the enemy," because we value life above almost all else. But death is an enemy we cannot defeat in this world. So we fight a battle we know cannot be won.

physician, the challenge is to know when to accept responsibility, and when to understand that a patient not taking responsibility does not mean that the physician has failed.

When I first saw the Murillo painting in London in 2010, it was a critical time for me in many ways. A number of changes were occurring in my life, and after years of never really being able to get away from it all, and being unwilling to accept life on life's terms, the stress was building and my resilience was fading. I was slipping into a depression that I could not see coming, and the severity of which others did not recognize since the symptoms I exhibited externally did not truly reveal what I was experiencing internally. The guidelines of the Substance Abuse and Mental Health Services Administration (SAMHSA) state that "because numbing symptoms hide what is going on inside emotionally, there can be a tendency for family members, counselors, and other behavioral health staff to assess levels of traumatic stress symptoms and the impact of trauma as less severe than they actually are."[62] Ultimately, I was diagnosed with post-traumatic stress disorder (PTSD) associated with that depression.[63]

The past I never dealt with was catching up to me. I, however, was not catching up to me. I was so afraid of my worthlessness being discovered (toxic shame) that I used perfection and control as a way to avoid my feelings. That façade of control, in a very real sense, was my addiction. I came into treatment thinking I wasn't an addict or alcoholic, kind of like the guy who thinks he is the only innocent person in prison. I was in prison, but it was one I had built myself. I

---

62   Loretta Malta et al., "Correlates of Functional Impairment in Treatment-Seeking Survivors of Mass Terrorism," *Behavior Therapy* 40, no. 1 (April 2009), 39–49.

63   K. C. Koenen et al., "Early Childhood Factors Associated with the Development of Post-Traumatic Stress Disorder: Results from a Longitudinal Birth Cohort," *Psychological Medicine* 37, no. 2 (February 2007), 181–192; Norah C. Feeny et al., "Exploring the Roles of Emotional Numbing, Depression and Dissociation in PTSD," *Journal of Traumatic Stress* 13, no. 3 (2000), 489–498.

had given up my rights as a human being. I had given up on how I was made. When I lost contact with my feelings, I also lost contact with my longings, needs, desires, and hope.

At the time, Evelyn and I felt our household emptying like water pouring out of a pitcher. Caleb, our youngest, was about to start high school just as our oldest son, Shawn, was finishing his junior year. Meanwhile, our daughter and eldest child, Rebecca, was spending a semester abroad at the University of London and living with a five centimeter thyroid mass—large for a thyroid nodule—which had been discovered in her right lobe just a few days before the beginning of the semester. A needle biopsy had indicated it was probably benign, so surgical removal would wait until the semester ended in June. At the same time, Evelyn's parents, and mine, were starting to have needs typical of people in their late sixties and early seventies: open heart surgeries, treatment for bladder cancer, a knee replacement, carotid artery surgery, abdominal aortic aneurysm surgery with a graft, and a host of other unassociated minor issues.

As medical professionals who have been in western Kentucky for more than two decades—Evelyn is a dermatologist with a solo wellness center and skin care practice; I am senior partner of an ENT practice—we are often casually approached by people wanting medical advice. Interestingly, many people seem to be of the opinion that physicians are always on duty. There may be some truth in that. After all, a medical emergency in midflight or in a public place often leads to the cry, "Is there a physician in the house?" But even stopping at the grocery store or trying to dine out, physicians may find themselves "at work." It is not uncommon for someone to roll up a sleeve, lift up a shirt, or even disrobe inappropriately in public to ask Evelyn about a rash, spot, or mole. Similarly, I am often stopped and asked about a child's sore throat or ear infection, or an adult's sinus or allergy issues.

So, leaving town on vacation is good for us; it gives us a chance to try to be "normal" people for a few days. However, early in a physician's career, or for those in private practice, even leaving town is not always a getaway. For a time, I had a solo practice during which vacations were never really getaways at all. For instance, I recall standing in line at Walt Disney World's Space Mountain and calling in a prescription for eardrops for a child. While on "vacation" I have prescribed antibiotics, discussed follow-up care with emergency doctors, spoken with oncologists about surgery timing for patients with head and neck cancer, and taken phone calls about patients who had died.

During my fifteen-year stint as medical director of an ambulatory surgery center, I dealt with a host of administrative burdens during "vacations," including coverage withdrawal by the affiliated hospital's anesthesia group the day before a vacation with extended family. We took the trip in spite of that last-minute crisis, but I spent much of my time on the phone arranging for coverage. Of course, as it is with some family vacations, a number of medical calamities also occurred during that trip—my daughter's frightening bicycle wreck, an ER visit for Evelyn in the middle of the night, and sons who, it seemed, were always vomiting for some reason or another.

Often, it seems that no matter how much time a physician spends "working" while on "vacation," it is not uncommon to return to a backlog of reports, lab tests, and patients with urgent needs. It is easy to question whether leaving is worth the trouble, considering how much the work seems to multiply while the physician is out. Still, it is better for the physician—and family—in the long run. A few days away can do a world of good to replenish the spirit.

The bottom line is that it is all about establishing appropriate boundaries and abiding by them. It can be difficult to recognize and admit the stress that results from the type of 24/7/365 commitment that the job seems to dictate. Yet it can also be difficult to understand that it is critical for physicians to carve out some "sacred space" for themselves, and for others to understand the need for that space, and to respect it. Peabody's obiter dictum[64] has been appropriately broadened: "The secret of the care of the patient *is caring for oneself* while caring for the patient" (emphasis added).[65]

PAIN: TRANSFORM OR TRANSMIT

When I returned to the Murillo painting at the National Gallery in the early summer of 2016, I was in a much different place from the one when I first saw the masterpiece. Evelyn and I had come to London to visit friends, and I was eager to see "my paintings" again.

The bottom line is that it is all about establishing appropriate boundaries and abiding by them. It can be difficult to recognize and admit the stress that results from the type of 24/7/365 commitment that the job seems to dictate. Yet it can also be difficult to understand that it is critical for physicians to carve out some "sacred space" for themselves, and for others to understand the need for that space, and to respect it.

---

64   Francis Peabody, "The Care of the Patient," *Journal of the American Medical Association* 88, no. 12 (March 19, 1927), 877–882.

65   Lucy Candib, *Medicine and the Family: A Feminist Perspective* (New York: Basic Books, 1995).

When I entered the gallery where it was displayed, the Murillo was to my right and a little behind me. When I turned to look at it, I was so close that its size and scale again took me aback; for a moment, I was mesmerized. Then I felt immense, unexpected waves of emotion—sadness, hurt, and gladness swept over me. I began to weep unashamedly, abundant tears streaming down my cheeks. I then felt Evelyn's hand gently touch the small of my back as she joined me in weeping in silence. After twenty-nine years of marriage, nothing needed to be said. She knew better than anyone the pain associated with my journey. She had lived it with me; I had allowed my hurt and loneliness and bitterness of spirit to wound her many times over. I was, in many respects, like the paralytic in that I was by the pool as a result of my own "doings."

Fr. Richard Rohr has written, "If we do not transform our pain, we will most assuredly transmit it."[66] The natural inclination for many people is to bury their pain and suffering and forget it. After all, what good is accomplished by dredging up the past? What sense does it make to relive painful events, failures, and misdeeds, and to commiserate about trauma suffered? Unfortunately, the world is full of people who think they bury their pain, only to turn around and transmit it.[67]

But, as civil rights leader Mahatma Gandhi said, "An eye for an eye makes the whole world blind." It seems there is a demarcation between burying one's pain and absorbing it without reflecting or transmitting it. While the world catapults toward blindness, it is one thing to understand that the transformation of pain is necessary, but it is another thing to be able to accomplish it within oneself. That is

---

66   Richard Rohr, *Things Hidden: Scripture as Spirituality* (Cincinnati: Franciscan Media, 2008), 25.

67   Notable examples of transforming pain can be found in the work of KenyaRelief and Nate's Wish.

one of the most vital functions of authentic, credible religion. When people recognize they are in need of a transformative experience, the real work can begin.

Murillo captures the moment when Jesus asks the question, "Do you want to be made well?" It seems a rather odd question to ask someone who has been waiting by a pool every day for a miracle, especially someone without much hope of a miracle. Who would choose to stay sick?

The fact is that a physician sees many people every day who would rather remain in their condition than change their life. The offer of a pill or a procedure—even a risky operation—is often received with greater appreciation and readiness of spirit than the admonition or recommendation to change behavior and be healed. I have had patients complain to my office manager and report negatively on patient satisfaction surveys because I have moved into difficult conversations regarding their weight, eating habits, alcohol intake, smoking—and the list goes on. Some have even remarked on surveys that I discussed things that were none of my business.

Jesus asks the question: Do you have the will necessary to be restored? According to the Roman philosopher Lucius Annaeus Seneca, the wish to be cured is part of the cure. You can sense the "paralytic's" exasperation in the painting, demonstrated by his outstretched arms, inviting a response from the Lord. He looks up with palms facing heavenward as if to say, "What more could I do? What more do you want from me? I would do anything to be made well. Don't you see?"

As Chip Dodd wrote, "We become experts at practicing hopelessness, not believing that our hearts' yearnings are real, denying that our feelings matter, and lacking the faith that we are really made as persons of immense value. We deny our innate wishes for more life and love."[68]

How can physicians get patients to do what they need to do when they are not interested in the type of healing that's needed? Sometimes patients think they want to get well, but they are expecting the angel to stir the water. Because the treatment offered is not what is expected, the opportunity for healing can go unrecognized.[69]

What is needed is a paradigm shift in thinking. Many people desire healing today, but they want and expect a surgery or a pill. They want healing, but only the way they want it; many of them reject the need to change themselves or their behavior. That is what I needed, a paradigm shift in my thinking.

FROM THE PARALYTIC'S POINT OF VIEW

How would you respond if you were to make yourself the paralytic? Have you ever made your own pleas to God, wondering what He was up to? Have you ever wondered if He sees you, lying in your own pool of despair?

I have wondered if He hears my prayers. I have wondered if He wandered by, aware that I was unable to alter my plight, aware that others were in line to receive the blessing of healing I needed. My soul has cried out, "I cannot do this! My life is unmanageable."

That is, essentially, what the paralytic confesses: utter powerlessness over his circumstances. That is exactly when healing appears for the man by the pool. And that is the moment when healing becomes accessible to us. It comes when you can admit to being powerless, when you can dare to admit that your life has become unmanage-

---

68   Chip Dodd, *The Voice of the Heart: A Call to Full Living*, 2nd ed. (Nashville: Sage Hill Resources, 2014), 17.

69   II Kings 5 relates the story of just such a man.

able. When you become the paralytic—disabled by your own pool of despair—that is when the healing can begin. That is when you can see yourself for who you are.

CALLED TO DO HIS WORK

When I dare to place myself in the painting as Jesus, I feel an immense responsibility to lend that hand, to try and elevate my fellow man, to be a conduit of healing. That is, on some level, the role of the physician. Physicians have some sort of duty to society that is generally implicitly acknowledged as a result of having gone to medical school and completed training. An empathic concern or compassion for my patients' situations and a desire to alleviate their suffering is what they deserve and how I best serve.

However, there is also a sense that our responsibility is qualitatively, if not quantitatively, different from the responsibility of a lawyer, an electrician, an accountant, or any other professional. Emily Lu, a medical student, concluded that our obligation demands that we "deeply respect the fact that every patient, when they come to us, has entrusted us with their bodies and their lives."[70] That level of trust carries with it an enormous burden.

Terminally ill neurosurgeon Paul Kalanithi poignantly wrote about this in his memoir, *When Breath Becomes Air*. Discussing whether or not being a physician was worth the cost, he felt it was the encounters with patients and their families that were the reward. But he also admitted these rewards came at a very high emotional cost. "The call to protect life ... was obvious in its sacredness," he noted. "The cost of my dedication to succeed was high, and the ineluctable

---

70 Emily Lu, "The 'Exceptional' Social Contract of Being a Physician," *Medicine for Change* (blog), September 12, 2010, accessed June 16, 2017, blog.emily.lu/ physician-social-contract/.

failures brought me nearly unbearable guilt. Those burdens are what make medicine holy and wholly impossible: in taking up another's cross, one must sometimes get crushed by the weight."[71]

Kalanithi's inner drive, I believe, was deeper than the typical definition of success. He was driven to succeed with every patient, in every circumstance—every operation, every needle stick, every decision, everything. Hence, the crushing weight that comes by carrying that cross. He spoke of an inner demon I can hardly bring myself to name when I am dealing with people's lives. That demon is perfection.

The cross of perfection is a cross that the Lord has never asked anyone to carry. It is a tortuous dance of imprisonment that many physicians, many surgeons, eagerly embrace. Yet, I not only have attempted to pick it up; I have actually imagined myself carrying it. I want to do the work of Jesus. I just can't be Jesus and, sometimes, I hate myself for it. In order to compensate for my own contempt of my humanity and the attendant limitations associated with it, I developed an insufferable air of arrogance. This act hides my shame and my fear that I am an imposter. And I am not alone. In fact, there is an old riddle that is humorous only to the extent that it encapsulates this idea:

Q: What is the difference between God and a surgeon?
A: God doesn't think He is a surgeon.

A PHYSICIAN'S LIFE—NOT NECESSARILY FAMILY FRIENDLY

The demands on a physician's time, energy, intellect, emotional well-being, and family are unique.

---

71   Paul Kalanithi, *When Breath Becomes Air* (New York: Random House, 2016), 98.

Looking at the Murillo painting, my thoughts turn to my children. The demands on medical families can border on rigorous, ludicrous, inappropriate, suffocating, appreciated, overlooked, applauded, pitied, and expected—all at the same time. What has it meant for my children to have two parents who are physicians?

One day when my daughter, Rebecca, was at a summer scholarship program during her high school years, she called me wanting medical advice for a friend. "Dad, one of the girls up here has some really bad nasal congestion that is getting worse. What would you do?" I first told her it would be hard to say without an examination, and then I told her to try some over-the-counter decongestants and perhaps an antihistamine. If that didn't work, I said I'd probably prescribe a couple of nasal sprays. "I've already done all that," she said. "What would you do next?" That's when it dawned on me that her peers held the notion that she was somehow imbued with a thorough and innate knowledge of medicine, and she had not only accepted that notion but acted on it. There she was, prescribing medication while away from home—and she wasn't even on vacation.

Around age three, my oldest son, Shawn Jr., was enamored with his telephone pull-toy. One evening while we were preparing dinner he picked up the phone unprompted and screamed into the receiver, "Patient! I thought I told you never to call me at home!" He then abruptly slammed down the receiver and walked away. Evelyn and I looked at each other in disbelief, each of us promptly denying we had ever acted that way. We concluded he must have witnessed the behavior at a physician-friend's house, and surmised that he probably just got things a little out of order. After all, he was only three. Clearly, Evelyn and I would have taught him to slam down the phone first, wait for it to disconnect, and then scream into the harmless receiver.

After Caleb, our youngest, had braces applied to his teeth, I came home after work one day to find him in a significant amount of discomfort. He asked me to take a look at his mouth, where I found quite a few swollen, but superficial ulcers on the buccal mucosa and tongue. "Wow, Caleb," I said. "I am very sorry. That looks like it really hurts." Just as I was about to offer recommendations for relief, he interrupted me and, as though speaking to a stranger, softly asked, "Dad? That is almost like—compassion?" All I could do was laugh, cry, and hug him. I suspect it is not easy being the son of a surgeon.

In many ways, this life of a physician is not worth it. Often, students enter medical school as caring, compassionate people with an innate desire to serve and offer themselves in doing so. Somehow the process of becoming a physician and practicing as a surgeon drives much of that passion for life and for their work out of them, and leaves them with little compassion for themselves or for others. While there is an argument to be made that I succumbed to burnout because of some inherent defect or weakness, the staggering figures suggest that there are structural, organizational, even systemic problems in the process of training and practicing that deserve investigation and redress. Identifying and enhancing the tools available for individual physicians to increase resilience and decrease stress to mitigate burnout is necessary, but *not* sufficient.

The painting demonstrates that there is a hand reaching out to help. The healing needed is available, though it often does not come in the form or timing of the demands—just as it did not for the paralytic.

The work for physicians struggling through the healing journey is to be willing to admit their own powerlessness, to recognize and even embrace their neediness, their humanity. By letting go of that facade of control and perfection that someone may think they possess—that they may even believe that they need—they gain access to all they need, and often all that they want. You can aspire to be a healer and do His work without pretending to be perfection incarnate.

WHAT HAPPENS IN PROCESS GROUP, STAYS IN PROCESS GROUP

*One of the most challenging—translation: **fear-inducing**—parts of my CPE experience was a group session called Process Group. I did not attend Process Group for the first couple of weeks because I had a full schedule of individual sessions with different counselors. I suppose I needed, initially, a lot of attention and therapy for my "brain dead" state.*

During that time, I would hear occasional rumblings about something that had happened in Process Group, but there was a standing guideline that "what happens in Process Group, stays in Process Group." That's a tough guideline for a bunch of addicts living together without anything with which to medicate themselves. It was doubly tough for me because it was something out of my control, something unfamiliar, which intensified my fear going into my first Process Group.

We were instructed to sit in a tight circle of chairs, so close that our knees were touching. The process itself was relatively scripted, with a few rules thrown in. The counselor would ask who wanted to start, to which someone would reply, for example: "I have a confrontation for Shawn." I was to answer, "Okay, Stan, what's your confrontation?" He would then voice an issue or problem that occurred recently that involved me, with the only rule being that he had to also offer a little of himself. So, he couldn't get away with saying, "You always take all the hot water before I can shower." Instead, he would have to also share his feelings on the matter: "I feel anger, sadness, and some hurt when you take all the hot water." After this he would have to expand on those emotions. I would be expected to respond by first thanking him for telling me of his feelings about the incident, and then stating how I felt in return. Rationalization, defending, blaming, explaining was not allowed.

*What is really crazy is how absolutely hyped-up and scared to death I was to be in a room with a group of men talking about things I had been trying to avoid all of my life: feelings. I was abjectly terrified. And **wow**, it was unbelievable to discover that my first impulse was to explain, justify, and defend.*

It took a while, but I really started to like Process Group. I was coming to really know other men while discovering some of myself. It was powerful stuff, scary, but powerful stuff.

FIND YOUR
HEART

As you examine your own situation, remember these points:

- Admit your wound and your need for help.

- Establish boundaries: professional, personal, and emotional.

- Develop a language to express your feelings. Then express them honestly with someone you can trust, as scary as that feels. Consider reading Chip Dodd's *Voice of the Heart.*

- Transform your pain. This requires a spiritual practice.

Ask yourself these questions to help you begin your own healing journey:

- Visiting or comforting the sick is one of the seven corporal acts of mercy. "Instructing, advising, consoling, comforting are spiritual works of mercy," according to the catechism of the

Catholic Church.[72] Do you think of your work as merciful? What either prompts or inhibits you from viewing your work as merciful? Could you come to see your work as an extension of mercy? How would that make you feel?

▫ Does your work reflect the actions of instruction, advice, consolation, and comfort on a daily basis? How does this awareness encourage you? Harm you? Possibly encourage your patients? Harm them?

---

72 *Catechism of the Catholic Church*, 2nd ed. (Washington, DC: United States Conference of Bishops, 2000, 2016), 588.

FOUR

THE DEAD CHRIST: THE STORY OF THE INTIMATE FRIEND

What the caterpillar calls disaster, the Master calls a butterfly.

—Cynthia Bourgeault

Philippe de Champaigne painted *Le Christ mort couché sur son linceul* (*The Dead Christ Lying on His Shroud*) around 1654. He graphically portrays a moment alluded to in the following passage from Luke's narrative to Theophilus:[73]

> Now behold, there was a man named Joseph, a council member, a good and just man. He had not consented to their decision and deed. He was from Arimathea, a city of the Jews, who himself was also waiting for the kingdom of God. This man went to Pilate and asked for the body of Jesus. Then he took it down, wrapped it in linen, and laid it in a tomb that was hewn out of the rock, where no one had ever lain before. That day was the Preparation, and the Sabbath drew near.

---

73   Luke 23:50–54. Parallel passages include Matthew 27:57–61, Mark 15:42–47, and John 19:38–42 (New King James Version).

Following my freshman year of medical school at the University of Louisville, I chose to do a rotation through various specialties in a community hospital as part of the Medical Education Community Orientation (MECO) program. MECO was an effort to expose big-city medical students to smaller community facilities and practices.

My rotation was for eight weeks at King's Daughter's Hospital in my hometown, Frankfort, Kentucky. I was given a stipend for the eight-week summer stint, but I would have done it for nothing. The rotation allowed me to follow a different local physician each week in addition to observing pretty much everything in the hospital. So, for instance, while following an internist, I might be called to the emergency room or a physician's office to observe a particularly interesting patient. Since the hospital was so small, and rarely had medical students in attendance, the physicians and nurses were always on the lookout for something to share with me. It was a tremendous experience, and a perfect complement to my studies in biochemistry, physiology, embryology, anatomy, and histology. Every morning I woke up at six o'clock excited to go to work, and I stayed there until late into the night. I loved it.

One morning the cardiologist I was shadowing told me he had something for me to do. Randy Schell was a young cardiologist, just a few years out of residency, but in the short time I had spent with him, I had already esteemed him to be a good physician. He was astute, thoughtful, and an effective communicator, taking the time to help the uninitiated—me—understand the intricacies of various issues. He embodied the type of doctor I was always drawn to throughout my residency, the kind who was an intellectual but who also cared as much about medical students and residents as they did about their patients.

As we waited for the elevator that morning, he looked at me with a wondering, remote scrutiny. When a smile crept slowly across his face, I asked him, "What's wrong?"

"I was just wondering where my twenties went," he replied, wryly shaking his head. "Spent in a library, I suppose." The elevator door opened and we stepped in.

A few minutes later, we reached our destination floor, exited the elevator, and headed to the nurse's station where we gathered the chart for a patient he had admitted the night before. It was a very clinical description: An eighty-seven-year-old man with end-stage heart disease S/P MI in the remote past. Patient had a stroke three months prior. He had been in a nursing home since that time gradually deteriorating. His kidneys stopped working the day before and he became obtunded.

"Go over his labs and x-rays, and I'll be back in a few minutes," Randy said.

In looking over the reports, I found that—other than labs that indicated the man had minimal renal function—there was nothing else in his chart. There was nothing to indicate that any workup had been done to try to determine to what extent his cardiac disease was contributing to his kidney failure, or if it was primarily renal in origin. There was no CT scan to examine his brain for any new infarction or stroke.

"What do you think?" Randy asked on his return. Confused, I hesitated to reply right away. I had not been a medical student very long, but I already knew that questioning authority clinically in a situation like the one I was in was fraught with hazard.

"Well," I cautiously ventured, "we haven't done an adequate renal, neuro, or cardiac workup, so I think I would start with his—"

"Living will," Randy interjected. "Good. Follow me."

We walked down the hallway and entered the man's room. He lay uncovered on the bed with one leg off the edge. Randy motioned to me to help him and together we straightened the man up in bed and covered him. Then Randy looked me in the eyes, turned away from the bed, and whispered to me so the patient could not possibly hear, "Have you ever seen anyone die?"

"No," I replied.

"Okay," he said. "I want you to sit down in the chair there. It's time you become acquainted with death. As physicians, we should be acquainted with death, but I never saw anyone die until late in medical school. I believe this gentleman is going to die today, and I think you should watch him do it. He doesn't have any family, so no one will be visiting. Call me when he dies, and then you can catch up with me."

Then he turned and left the room.

I sat in the corner of the room in an awkward chair that was designed to look relatively comfortable and inviting, but was neither. Cell phones and tablets had not been invented yet, so there was nothing to do but watch the patient.

For a little over two hours, the only sound in the room was his breathing. It had a crescendo-decrescendo cadence to it, punctuated by periods when he did not breathe at all. Gradually as his breathing grew abnormally deeper and faster, and those periods without breath appeared to lengthen, I realized he was experiencing Cheyne-Stokes respiration, also known as the death rattle.

I felt I was a voyeur. There I was, alone, watching him at a very intimate moment, which I had no right to witness. For a moment, I was aware of what an agonizing experience it was for me. Then my thoughts turned to him, his life, his hopes, his dreams. What had he accomplished? What had he had left undone? Who in his life had died before him? Had he outlived everyone in his life? Or had he become estranged from them through living?

His punctuated breathing continued. I thought about my own demise. What might I be thinking in my last moments of life? Would I be incapacitated and unaware? Would my death be a painful, lengthy demise from a malignancy, ALS/Lou Gehrig's disease, or some other disease? Would I be mowing the yard at forty-eight years old and have a massive heart attack, never even knowing death was imminent?

The man's breathing continued. And I went on thinking of my own end. When would it come? Would I be in an automobile accident on the way home from the hospital? Would I make it home at the end of that very day?

I thought back to when I was ten years old and my father was a young trooper with the Kentucky State Police, he shared with me intimate details of an accident that had haunted him for years. I believe the fear and sadness that event caused in him compelled him to share those details with me. His sadness undoubtedly came from the senseless loss of life, and his fear was for me as I entered a potentially dangerous period in life. The accident was a particularly gruesome automobile wreck involving four teenagers who died on impact with a pine tree on a curve their car had failed to negotiate. My father was one of the first responders, and as part of the accident investigation he had to take pictures of the scene. He showed the photos to me—something I would never "un-see." He wanted to impress on me the consequences of drinking, driving, speeding, and recklessness. If he wanted me to be haunted by those pictures as he and my mother were, his plan worked. Job's friend Bildad called death the "king of terrors."[74] I agree.

74   Job 18:14.

My mind returned to the man lying in the bed. His breathing seemed shallower. Or was it? I felt a twinge of guilt. Desiring my ordeal to be over meant desiring his life's end. For a moment, I felt compelled to hold his hand. But I resisted. His breathing began to slow and become even shallower. That went on for what seemed like an eternity; it was maybe three minutes.

His respiratory rate slowed to the point where I honestly thought it was over. Suddenly he let out a small sigh, and took another breath. He stopped breathing two or three times. He sighed again and took another breath. I held his hand.

Then he was gone.

Over the years, I have been transported back to that bedside many times. I have since seen many people take their last breath.

Randy Schell taught me about the sanctity of life in allowing me to witness death for the first time. It was an introduction that needed to be made. For death is the enemy of a physician, but an enemy that is to be respected if for no other reason than because, eventually, everyone will meet death.

DISCOVERING THE PAINTING

It is better to go to the house of mourning, than to go to the house of feasting: for that is the end of all men; and the living will lay it to heart.

—Ecclesiastes 7:2

One of our family traditions is a college graduation trip. Evelyn and I promised our children that upon completion of a four-year degree, father-son or mother-daughter would travel essentially anywhere the graduate wanted to go. We thought it would be a good opportunity for quality one-on-one time with each child while celebrating the accomplishment. For Rebecca's graduation, she and Evelyn went to Austria. When Shawn's graduation approached, the travel options had been narrowed to hiking the Incan Trail and visiting Machu Picchu, or following the World War II Normandy-to-Berchtesgaden path of the 101st Airborne. Both ideas sounded fabulous to me, but ultimately Shawn ended up going to Peru during the fall, before graduation, as part of a resident Spanish course. He got to see Machu Picchu, and I got to see his pictures, and his trip meant that he and I would go to Europe.

After graduation, we flew to Paris, the first leg of the France, Holland, Belgium, and Bavaria tour. We went a few days early to take in the city, arriving in the morning after flying all night from Atlanta, Georgia. That day, we walked about twelve miles, taking in the sights, including the Eiffel Tower. I had always envisioned standing atop that renowned landmark with my beloved, but I never imagined the person I would do this first with would be my twenty-two-year-old son. We ate at multiple restaurants and visited Notre Dame and Sacre Coeur de Montmartre.

Having a huge desire to visit the Louvre as well as the Musée d'Orsay, but having limited time to do so, I enlisted the help of a private guide. In preparing for the trip, I had read that the Louvre's collection included Caravaggio's *Death of the Virgin*. I wanted to see it, along with the Louvre's popular pieces such as the *Venus de Milo*, the *Mona Lisa*, *Wedding at Cana*, and the *Winged Victory of Samothrace*.

When we arrived at the Louvre, our guide informed us that *Death of a Virgin* was in a separate exhibition that required an additional fee of twenty euros per person. She told us that it was not widely considered one of Caravaggio's best works and that there were "plenty of other things to see."

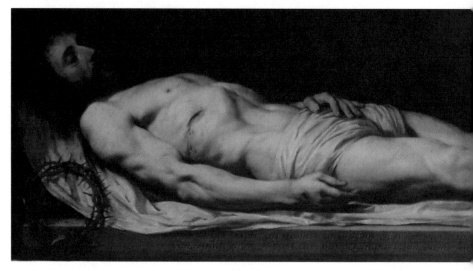

Le Christ mort couché sur son linceul (*The Dead Christ*), Philippe de Champaigne

Undeterred, I decided we would see it, having come so far. A voice inside me compelled me to do so. I believe that I need to listen to that small voice[75] when it speaks at such moments. Hearing that voice requires an inner quietness I have not always possessed, but I have slowly come to recognize and trust the power and veracity of His gentle whisper in guiding my heart. I usually find there is a reason for it that is not readily apparent.

When we entered the exhibition just off the gallery of the first floor, I immediately searched for the *Virgin*. It was close to the entrance, and, at one hundred forty-five by ninety-six inches, it was massive. Although it was beautiful and elegant in the same manner as other Caravaggios I had seen, it did not particularly move me. With only a few hours to explore the vast museum, I did not stop to ponder why I felt unmoved.

As I turned to walk away, I was transfixed by what caught my eye. Without even turning to look for him, I called to my son to

75   I Kings 19:12.

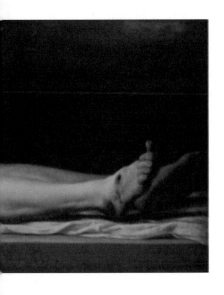

join me. "You have to see this," I said. We stood there gazing at Philippe de Champaigne's *Le Christ mort couché sur son linceul* (*The Dead Christ*). Its dimensions—two foot two by six foot five—were unusual but perfectly suited to the subject. It was displayed alone on a relatively short partition wall slightly below eye level, which increased the dramatic effect. My son and I stood there for several moments, neither of us speaking. It was a holy moment.

I tried to discern exactly what captivated me about the piece. From the standpoint of realism, Champaigne's interpretation is phenomenal. The anatomy alone is very good: a perfect representation of the imperfect human form. The figure is consistent with a thirty-year-old man in good shape, apparently murdered, the evidence being a slit-like wound in the right upper thorax, or chest. The marks of crucifixion are evident on the hands and feet.[76] The cloth underneath the body is reminiscent of the Shroud of Turin, or the Lirey Shroud. These both date to at least the fourteenth century and certainly would have been known to Champaigne, especially as a student of Nicolas Poussin, a French Baroque painter. The blood stains are evident on the edges of the burial cloth but are relatively subtle.

The figure's face is shadowed. The painting's dramatic contrasts of darkness and light (tenebrism) draw the observer's attention to the

---

76   William D. Edwards, Wesley J. Gabel, and Floyd E. Hosmer, "On the Physical Death of Jesus Christ," *Journal of the American Medical Association* 255, no. 11 (1986), 1455–1463.

body and its wounds. Blood appears to gently trickle from each of the wounds, implying that the death is recent, and the resurrection far away. Except for the blood, there is no hint of movement in the piece. Movement, typically, is a sign of life, but in this painting, paradoxically, the only movement is a sign of death. Almost as an afterthought, the crown of thorns lies propped just off the right shoulder of the ethereal corpse as if it had rolled off the head when the body was placed where it now lies.

My connection to the painting comes from a combination of emotions, particularly fear and loneliness. Fear of my own mortality and death draws me to identify with the dead Christ. Identifying with Him in repose, with death upon Him—as it will be for me one day—is much easier than identifying with Him in His righteousness as the Savior, someone who fed the five thousand, forgave the woman for her adultery, walked on water, died on the cross, ascended into heaven, and is seated at the throne. The painting screams aloneness to me, yet it is through that, coupled with fear, that I connect with Christ's humanity.

Aloneness and loneliness are difficult to escape for someone who always felt a bit like an only child—my sole sibling, my sister Beth, is thirteen years my junior. As with old friends, the feelings of aloneness and loneliness are such constant companions in my life that I easily dismiss them or fail to recognize their presence. There, on the mortuary slab, lying on His death shroud, I see Him in a place where we all lie alone—I see me in Him. In Him, I am alone; with Him, together. Seeing Him there on the canvas, I feel my aloneness most intensely. Yet at the same time, I feel most like Him, and therefore there is also a deep sense of togetherness.

Wisdom accompanies the emotions evoked by this painting. From the painting, I came to realize that intimacy and discernment arise from the acknowledgment that therein lies my destiny. Intimacy is the gift of loneliness. Wisdom is the gift of fear.[77] And the fear of the Lord is the beginning of wisdom.[78]

DEATH IS ALWAYS CLOSE IN MEDICINE

The first semester in medical school is punctuated by gross anatomy, which is more than just a course; it is a near-mythic rite of passage for aspiring physicians. It involves dissecting a human corpse, a body that not long before was a living being with hopes, dreams, aspirations, and loves, maybe with some of the same experiences you have had. Even with gloves, a shower, and a change of clothes, the formalin used to preserve the tissue for dissection follows you that first semester, reminding you of the lifeless body from which you are learning the intricacies, variations, and similarities of structure of the human form.

During dissection labs, there were a few instances when I found myself intently focused on an aspect of anatomy, only to suddenly realize how macabre the scene might look to a casual observer. Students wearing stained, white lab coats, scrubs, and gloves intensely studying dead bodies on a Saturday night when most twenty-two-year-olds are out doing anything else. From the high windows of a third-floor room, you could just make out the cars on I-65 cruising by, oblivious to the machinations in the large room full of corpses illuminated with fluorescent lights in an otherwise largely darkened building. The contrast between life, death, and life in the midst of death was palpable.

---

77   Chip Dodd, *The Voice of the Heart: A Call to Full Living*, 2nd ed. (Nashville: Sage Hill Resources, 2014), 66–107.

78   Proverbs 9:10.

There were four medical students to a cadaver. Phil was my lab partner. He was to become an orthopedic surgeon. Steve and John, our tandem pair, were a budding infectious disease physician and a nephrologist, respectively. During the third portion of the course, the lab manual called for a sagittal split of the head and neck. The upper torso had previously been severed from the lower trunk, and the brain had already been removed. Using what appeared to be a fairly regular saw, we were to divide the head into right and left halves down the middle of the forehead and nose between the eyes, splitting the oral cavity and mouth, throat, esophagus, and trachea. The cut would provide better access for study.

Up to that point, all four of us had been relatively eager participants and learners. I don't recall there being any real difference in willingness or ability to dissect between the two future internists (Steve and John) and the two budding surgeons (Phil and myself).

Yet every one of us balked on making that particular cut. But my own hesitation only lasted for a few seconds; seeing the hesitation by my other lab partners, I knew someone had to do it. I picked up the saw and, while Phil held on to the neck and shoulders, I began sawing through the cadaver, starting at the top of head.

We finished the lab after three or four hours and I went home to my apartment off lower Brownsboro Road. I was sitting at my desk studying Grant's *Atlas of Anatomy* when the morning's activities really sunk in. I started sobbing uncontrollably. I was grateful my roommate was out that evening.

In the midst of sobbing, I suddenly became ashamed of my emotions. When the late afternoon October sun streamed in through the sliding glass doors that led to our ground-floor patio and I realized it was a beautiful fall day, I had an epiphany. I realized I had been granted a distinct honor. Learning the intricacies of human anatomy and how they informed function and physiology was a profound privilege, which was not granted for my benefit, except to the extent that my work would benefit others and society. To whatever degree I failed in that exercise, I would fail in purpose. It was a truly sobering moment, a coming to consciousness.

The Dead Christ reminds me of those still, lifeless bodies from my gross anatomy days. As does the figure of Christ himself, so do those corpses continue to have an impact on me, even though they are long gone. The lessons learned from them come to me when I most need them.

Over the years, when I have been fortunate and engaged enough to be truly present, I have learned lessons in humility from death.[79] Just as God told Adam, "For dust you are, and to dust you shall return."[80] There is a sense in which dirt is my origin and my destiny.

NEVER FORGET WHO YOU ARE

When I neared the end of my residency in otolaryngology, my grandmother, Olean, was in her early eighties.[81] She had always been the spiritual stalwart of our family. Hemorrhaging profusely following

---

79   Humility is derived from the Latin root *humus* (earth; of the earth).

80   Gen. 3:19.

81   As a single mother, she had raised my mother and uncle while living with her parents in rural Muhlenberg County, Kentucky. When I was a child, I referred to my great grandparents as Big Mama and Shorty. Her name came from the fact that my mother called her mother Little Mama and the older woman living in the home with them was thus aptly referred to as Big Mama. This was long before Pearl Bailey and *The Fox and the Hound*. Shorty, you might guess, was small in stature. At age twenty, he had also lost a leg below the knee in a wagon accident. But what I remember most about him was his incredibly optimistic spirit. He smoked a pipe and constantly massaged the stump of his amputation with rubbing alcohol, all the while singing, "Rufus Rastas Johnson Brown, what you gonna do when the rent come 'round?" The smell of rubbing alcohol still reminds me of him.

the delivery of her son (my uncle) in late 1937, she said a simple prayer: "Lord, save my life and I will become a student of your Word and follow it the remainder of my life." She survived and kept her promise. When my parents wavered in their faith and ceased any pretense of religiosity, it was my grandmother who took me to church, faithfully. Her thoughts, actions, comments, and outlook in life was always informed by her spirituality.

When I was accepted to medical school, there was a reception for me in Frankfort that consisted of friends and family. I was the first in the family to attend and graduate from college, so acceptance to medical school was a big deal. At the party, she pulled me aside and whispered, "I am so proud of you. But I am more proud of who you are than what you have done. Never forget who you are."

It was great advice. And while I sincerely thought I knew what she meant, I also thought I knew who I was. Over time, however, I found it very difficult to know who I was, so it was pretty much impossible to forget what I did not know in the first place.

Over the years, whenever anyone in the family has needed medical advice, I have generally been whom they turned to, regardless of the fact that I am an ENT. In their eyes, I'm a doctor, that's all that matters.

One day, when my grandmother experienced increasing shortness of breath, I contacted her family physician, who prescribed medication for congestive heart failure. Over the next year, she worsened. One day, she felt as if she were suffocating. Filled with fear, I called her doctor again. After he had talked to me about the medical aspects of her care and promised to continue caring for her as he always had, he said softly, "You know, Shawn, someday she is going to die." I thought that was heartless and rude—and honest. He was merely trying to get me to understand the inevitability of the story; it was not going to have a happy ending. She was referred to an outstanding cardiologist in Louisville, Dr. Bob Goodin, who diagnosed her with a dysfunctional aortic valve. The problem was escalating relatively quickly, and at eighty-five, her options were not good. Without surgery, she would gradually decompensate[82] and die. With surgery, she stood a decent chance of dying of some other cause, arguably not too far in the future, considering her years.

After a consultation with Alan Lansing, an eminent cardiovascular and thoracic surgeon in Louisville, she decided to pursue the valve-replacement operation. Although the family thought I had talked her into it, the truth was that she was miserable and wanted to get better or be done with it all. The idea that she would have to deal with a gradually worsening sensation of suffocating was unthinkable to her, so her decision seemed like sound reasoning to me.

She sailed through the operation, and I felt confident that she would recover and get her life back. I visited her several times during the first two postoperative days at the private suburban hospital where she'd had the operation. On the third day, she was scheduled to leave the intensive care unit (ICU) and move to the floor. I finished early at the ENT clinic where I was a chief resident, and I decided to visit her for lunch. Before leaving, I stopped by the office to pick up a few reports before heading out to my car. While still in the clinic parking lot, I received a call from the hospital's ICU nurse, who asked me to come back immediately. But it was already too late. A branch of my grandmother's pulmonary artery had ruptured, and she bled to death in a few minutes.

---

82 A nice code word, or doctor speak, which in this context means "to suffocate." As doctors, we get to use words that obscure the meaning just a little so as to take the sting out of it. We do this with feelings as well, so fear becomes concern, anger becomes frustration. It removes us just a little from our hearts and, perhaps arguably, from the truth.

Had I not stopped by the ENT office, I would have been at her bedside when she passed, a fact that has haunted me to this day. I was there for a complete stranger—the dying man without a family, whose death was the first I had witnessed—but I had missed the chance to be there for someone I loved very deeply, someone who was the kindest soul I had ever known.

I was conflicted, but my grandmother had made her peace before the operation and had even asked me to speak at her funeral if she failed to survive. The truth is my grandmother would have died alone, even if I had been by her side. Death is a journey we all make alone.

A THOUSAND DEATHS

In *A Farewell to Arms,* the renowned author Ernest Hemingway wrote, "The coward dies a thousand deaths, the brave but one. ... [The man who first said that] was probably a coward[83] ... He knew a great deal about cowards but nothing about the brave. The brave dies perhaps two thousand deaths if he's intelligent. He simply doesn't mention them."

I have died a thousand metaphoric deaths. Perhaps I could have spared myself a few of those deaths if I had developed the courage or heart to actually suffer well through one or two of them. Because of my own intractable unwillingness to be fully present, I suffered more than was necessary. It is arguable that without my hardheadedness, or hardheartedness, my fall would not have been sufficiently far enough to awaken me from the worldly stupor in which I was immersed.

If I place myself on the shroud in Champaigne's masterpiece, what would I see? My gaze would still be drawn to the lifeless body

---

83   William Shakespeare wrote that line spoken by Julius Caesar in *Julius Caesar.*

and its fresh wounds oozing blood and contaminating everything beneath. But unlike Jesus's wounds, the majority of mine were self-inflicted. These self-inflicted wounds were perpetrated as a result of vows I had made to protect my heart from pain and suffering. My metaphoric wounds not being acknowledged are, then, like the Lord's. They are not bandaged, and there is no evidence of any "care" of them.

With wounds still hurting, still oozing, I found my "lifeless corpse" enrolled in psychotherapy. My case was a bit unusual in comparison to some of the other attendees, since my treatment was not mandated by the intervention of some governing board or agency. There had been no professional seminal event. My license was not restricted, nor would it be. My decision to enroll in a recommended six-week, intensive, outpatient treatment program was entirely voluntary. I later discovered that most of the other men in the program doubted that I would return after my three-day evaluation, since I was not being forced to undergo treatment. Only one, who later became a very dear friend, felt certain I would come in on my own.

Most of the men in the treatment facility were addicted to at least one substance. My addiction, as I would learn, was control. I was codependent, addicted to seeking approval. In my quest to feel better I kept believing that another title, office, book, degree, car, or bible study might ease the ache for life, an ache caused by my inability to admit that I desired full, authentic living. Despondent and depressed, I was unaware of my self-taught hopelessness. Suicide is just "an attempt to kill hope, to make the ache for real life stop,"[84] but even that did not seem like a solution. I was burned up, burned

---

84 Chip Dodd, *The Voice of the Heart: A Call to Full Living*, 2nd ed. (Nashville: Sage Hill Resources, 2014), 17.

out, twisted, and defeated. I needed a time out. I needed my wounds addressed and I could not do it alone. It was only when Evelyn finally confronted me that I was forced to face my own emotional dysfunction. I had been emotionally absent for a long time and it was getting worse. I just wasn't aware of it. She refused to watch and be a witness to me pursuing this path of self-destruction.

I thought I had already died in multiple ways, but I entered treatment not realizing that the dying I would need to do in order to have the life I wanted was still before me.

In his book, *New Seeds of Contemplation,* Theologian Thomas Merton wrote, "Every one of us is shadowed by an illusory person: a false self. We are not very good at recognizing illusions, least of all the ones we cherish about ourselves." Jungians might term Merton's "false self" the ego.

By the time I entered therapy, my ego, to some degree, had been laid aside. I had killed it, and it needed to be put to death. I knew I needed help, and I was at the point where I would take good orderly direction. What surgeon is enamored with the idea of not just doing psychotherapy but actually realizing they *need* psychotherapy? That part of my ego at least was gone. Coming to terms with that was a type of death, the wounds of which were just as evident as they are in Champaigne's rendering of Christ, the wounds that dribbled pride and arrogance, that unceasingly sought approval and external satisfaction, and more. The ego is the zombieland of the psyche. The process of dying, for the ego, is much like trying to kill a zombie—I put mine to death and still struggle to keep it from rising again.

In Luke 9:22–24, immediately following the feeding of the five thousand and Peter's confession, Jesus says, "The Son of Man must suffer many things, and be rejected by the elders and chief priests and scribes, and be killed, and be raised the third day." Then He said to the five thousand, "If anyone desires to come after Me, let him deny himself, and take up his cross daily and follow Me. For whoever desires to save his life will lose it, but whoever loses his life for My sake will save it." What does it mean to deny myself? What does it mean to lose my life?

It is reasonable to surmise that there was a glimpse of the reality of Jesus during his transfiguration before Peter, James, and John.[85] Years later, both John and Peter wrote of it, speaking of His glory.[86] On that mount, in that moment, the curtain was pulled back to reveal the true nature of Jesus. They saw who He truly was and it made a lasting impact on them. That was, in essence, Jesus's true self. Is it possible I can tease back a curtain and reveal my true self?

THE WOUNDS OF THE SERVANT

What do the wounds mean? In *The Wounded Healer*, theologian Henri Nouwen addresses what it means to be a minister in contemporary society. Though Nouwen was discussing those who look after spiritual concerns, there is little doubt that he also recognized the broader application of his search for meaning. The Greek word for minister or servant is *diakonos*. A physician certainly fits into the paradigm of a servant and, in some respects, is a type of priest of the body. In an attempt to make some sense out of the modern situation, Nouwen discusses a suffering world, a suffering generation, a suffering man, and a suffering minister. Through a process he describes as somewhat fragmented, he slowly comes to recognize the image of a wounded healer:

---

85   Matthew 17:1–8.

86   John 1:14; II Peter 1:16–18.

After all attempts to articulate the predicament of modern man, the necessity to articulate the predicament of the minister himself became most important. For the minister is called to recognize the sufferings of his time in his own heart and make that recognition the starting point of his service. Whether he tries to enter into a dislocated world, relate to a convulsive generation or speak to a dying man, his service will not be perceived as authentic unless it comes from a heart wounded by the suffering about which he speaks.

Thus nothing can be written about ministry without a deeper understanding of the ways in which the minister can make his own wounds available as a source of healing.[87]

> *There is a great propensity for physicians to feel compelled to pose and pretend they're perfect, as if they have all the answers. That takes a lot of effort and energy. Do not be afraid to show your own humanity, your own wounds. That is the essence of being vulnerable. It is the ultimate sacrifice to place one's ego on the altar, but the wounds revealed in that demise are a source of healing for us and those we treat. We have the opportunity in that sense to do the work of Jesus in that His wounds are a source of healing for us spiritually.*

Empathy is the capacity to understand and/or feel what another is experiencing from within that person's frame of reference. In other

---

87   Henri Nouwen, *The Wounded Healer* (New York: Doubleday, 1979), xvi.

words, it is the capacity to place yourself in another's shoes. For clarity, I do not believe it is necessary that I suffer from the same malady I'm treating in order to have empathy for my patient. I do not need to have intimate knowledge of what it means to suffer diabetes in order to treat a diabetic appropriately, and with empathy. However, I do believe it is absolutely essential that I be in touch with my own humanity. I also believe it is critical that I be able to adequately express myself emotionally to truly be empathetic. If I am not in touch with my own feelings, it is impossible for me to be perceptive about yours in a meaningful way. Theory of mind, in other words, requires adequate interoceptive abilities. To engage as a doctor in a physician-patient relationship is to enter territory reserved for the courageous, or for those "with heart."

The French word for heart, *coeur*, is the root of the English word *courage*. When people talk about not losing heart, they're talking about courage. I believe this definition of courage is about keeping the heart open, because to keep the heart open in the face of fear, hurt, loneliness, and sadness takes great courage. In order to demonstrate empathy, one must have the courage to be in possession of the heart. It is logical and defensible to close down a little or a lot when subjected to an assault against the heart. But that self-protection comes with consequences. I made vows to myself to never suffer "like that" again. These vows I did my best to keep, and I suffered for it.

Those without heart are impaired in their ability to function in the health care environment. Without emotional competence, the heart has no voice, and the physician lacks the ability to empathize adequately with the patient. The situation can be approached intellectually—this is what the patient must be feeling, you might think—but without empathy, you are putting your patient, the relationship with your patient, and yourself at risk.

The professional hazards of attempting to function as a doctor without heart is similar to entering combat without a weapon. You may survive, but the odds are decidedly against you. When I think of classmates, friends in residency, or colleagues in practice, I am astonished by how many have been incapacitated or have been to treatment for alcoholism, drug addiction, depression, or anxiety.

> *The situation can be approached intellectually—this is what the patient must be feeling, you might think—but without empathy, you are putting your patient, the relationship with your patient, and yourself at risk.*

It is even more devastating to think of those who have taken their own lives out of hopelessness and despair. The paradox is in the recognition that hope lies in death. As a physician, when things look grim, I often say to patients and their family, "Where there is life, there is hope." But it is just as true that where there is death there is hope. Just as, for Christians, the hope of transformation lies in a dead Christ—because only a crucified Christ can rise on the third day—the hope of transformation, for all of us, lies in the death of the false self. That hope waits in pregnant anticipation of the relinquishment of the facade of control, programs for happiness, and unwillingness to not just be human but also embrace humanity.

There is so much fear and loneliness wrapped up in the perfectionism that I have demanded of myself and that has been projected upon me as a physician and a human being. As was the servant of Isaiah 53:5 called to suffer, I too am called to suffer in my service: "the chastisement of our peace was upon him; and with His stripes we are healed." As the Messiah's wounds became a source of healing, so too will my wounds.

However, your wounds are a source of healing for you as well as for those whom you've had the privilege to care. But you must address your own wounds. You must admit your woundedness, even though doing so is like death to you. It is in acknowledging your weakness, your frailty, and your faults that you become empowered to heal because you have embraced your humanity—out of which can arise your empathic true self. You have heart again. You are free to be you.

Imagine your image imposed upon the painting of Champaigne's dead Christ. What are your wounds? Do they feel fresh? Are they still oozing? Who is responsible for them? Who in your life is able to treat them? Are you a little surprised that you have been asked to make what feels like the ultimate sacrifice?

MY DEATH WOUND: MY STORY OF THE INTIMATE FRIEND

In a sense, I was dead in therapy. I had nothing. From the smallest to the largest things, from the dearest to the most trivial—everything was gone. In essence, it was just me alone in a strange place with people I either did not know at all or had met just a few weeks before. I had become acquainted with some of the other men in treatment during my three-day evaluation, but since I actually entered treatment a few weeks later, several of them had finished their three months of rehab and gone home, only to be replaced by a new guys.

The CPE guidelines dictated that no one could go anywhere alone. We ate together, went to the park together (usually on Saturdays), and attended church together on Sunday mornings. Every day we attended an AA meeting, sometimes during the day, sometimes at night, but nevertheless, every day. We drove from the apartments where we stayed to the CPE every morning and returned every afternoon following the day's treatment activities. I was not able to drive until they let me. I could call home once a week on a land line. I had a few books, including a Bible. But I had no computer, cell phone, patients, surgery schedule, room to myself, or anyone asking my opinion. In short, it was no life as I had known it. I was very lonely, but oddly comfortable there.

*Looking back on that time, there was also a deep relief or gladness beneath the fear and loneliness I experienced. I was hemmed in, but unshackled; dead, but sensing life just around the corner. It was almost as if I were young and happy again. In his book **The Things They Carried**, author Tim O'Brien describes perfectly what it is like to write about that time in my life: It is like "skimming across the surface of my own history, moving fast ... and when I take a high leap in the dark and come down ... years later, I realize it is as [Shawn] trying to save [Shawn's] life with a story."*[88]

FIND YOUR
HEART

- □ Surrendering to how we are made can feel like a type of death. How and in what situations have you surrendered your will? What did you learn from these experiences?

- □ Describe the difference between disaster and a butterfly while considering the quote at the beginning of the chapter: *What the caterpillar calls disaster, the Master calls a butterfly.*

---

88 Tim O'Brien, *The Things They Carried* (New York: Broadway Books, 1990), 246.

- What are the tools God utilizes to shape us in life? Consider Joseph,[89] Job,[90] Paul,[91] and the Syrophoenician woman.[92]

- In the "Find Your Heart" section at the end of the first chapter, you were asked to write about the five most painful events in your life and vows you may have made as a result. Review your writing about those events.

---

89 Genesis 37–50, with attention to 50:20.

90 Job 1, 39–42.

91 Acts 9.

92 Matthew 15:21–28.

FIVE

THE INCREDULITY OF SAINT THOMAS: THE STORY OF THE WOUND

Let a teacher wave away the flies and put a plaster on the wound. Don't turn your head. Keep looking at the bandaged place. That's where the light enters you. And don't believe for a moment that you're healing yourself.

—Rumi

About three or four years after the members of my family began training in taekwondo together, we each earned a black belt. It had been my idea to become involved in the activity in the first place, and most of the family was done with martial arts after earning black belts. Other sports were starting to take up more time, and it just seemed like everyone needed a break.

I, of course, was the exception. I was committed to working toward my second-degree belt. My daughter, Rebecca, was about eleven-years-old at the time, and for several months she dutifully went with me to the classes. One evening as she and I were getting ready to leave the house, Evelyn called me aside and said, "Honey, she doesn't want to go. Please don't make her go."

"I haven't made her go a single time," I replied somewhat indignantly. "I just ask her if she wants to go, and she always does."

"Ask her again, and give her permission to say no," Evelyn said.

"Fine," I replied. I walked into the family room, irritated at the implication. Rebecca was standing there with her jacket on, ready to leave. But I asked her, "Sweetheart, do you want to go to taekwondo with me tonight?"

"Yes, Daddy," she replied.

I felt much more confident that I was right about her desire, but just to prove it, I asked, "Are you sure? Daddy really wants to know the truth. I don't want you to go if you don't want to go."

With a huge grin on her face, Rebecca said, "Daddy if you want to go, I want to go with you." *How sweet is that?* I thought. Then she continued, "But if you don't ever want to go to taekwondo another time in your life, that would be okay with me, too."

I laughed and gave her a huge hug. I was very grateful for Evelyn's insight into my daughter's heart, but I was also sad and incredulous that I could be so blind to her desire. Somehow I had given her the message that her worth to me was tied to her participation in an activity I enjoyed. She was doing what she knew would please me, but denying her truth to do it.

I had, unfortunately, taught her well. She was codependent with me, afraid that if she expressed herself, I would abandon her. She denied her own feelings, needs, longings, and desires to please me. In that, regrettably, she lost herself.

THE PAINTING AND ITS PURPOSE

Being unwilling or unable to believe something is to be in a state of incredulity. *Merriam-Webster's* also defines incredulity as a withholding or refusal of belief; skepticism; unbelief; disbelief. With respect to issues of biblical faith, there is no state of being "unable to believe"—that situation simply does not exist. Unbelief is always a reflection of unwillingness. Mark 3 and Matthew 12 cite a sin that cannot be forgiven. Unwillingness is considered by many to be the key element in that type of transgression, a concept that fits well with the statement of Jesus in John 8:24: "I said therefore unto you, that ye shall die in your sins: for if ye believe not that I am He, ye shall die in your sins."

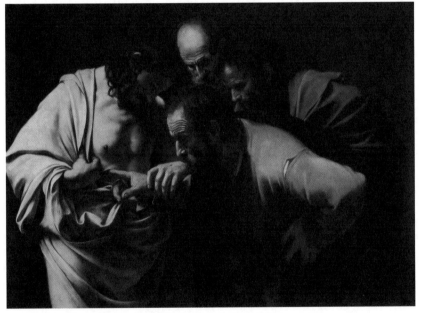

The Incredulity of Saint Thomas, Michelangelo Merisi da Caravaggio

Michelangelo Merisi da Caravaggio's painting, *The Incredulity of Saint Thomas,* c. 1603, depicts a scene from the gospel story following the resurrection of Christ. The episode is recorded in John 20:30. The action immediately precedes the statement of purpose John had in writing his gospel—namely, that it might produce belief.

Caravaggio's use of light in contrast to darkness reflects the spirit of the apostle John's writing. In John 1:5–6, for example, the apostle writes, "God is light, and in Him is no darkness at all. If we say that we have fellowship with Him, yet walk in darkness, we lie and do not practice the truth."

Understanding John's purpose in writing the story of Thomas—and Caravaggio's purpose in depicting it as he did—begins by reading John 20:19–31, and then taking some time to simply reflect on its meaning in Caravaggio's work. Be patient, and be sure to pay attention not just to the painting overall or its details but also to what the image stirs deep within you.

> Then, the same day at evening, being the first day of the week, when the doors were shut where the disciples were assembled for fear of the Jews, Jesus came and stood in the midst, and said to them, "Peace be with you." When He had said this, He showed them His hands and His side. Then the disciples were glad when they saw the Lord.
>
> So Jesus said to them again, "Peace to you! As the Father has sent Me, I also send you." And when He had said this, He breathed on them, and said to them, "Receive the Holy Spirit. If you forgive the sins of any, they are forgiven; if you retain the sins of any, they are retained."
>
> Now Thomas, called the Twin, one of the twelve, was not with them when Jesus came. The other disciples therefore said to him, "We have seen the Lord."
>
> So he said to them, "Unless I see in His hands the print of the nails, and put my finger into the print of the nails, and put my hand into His side, I will not believe."

And after eight days His disciples were again inside, and Thomas with them. Jesus came, the doors being shut, and stood in the midst, and said, "Peace to you!" Then He said to Thomas, "Reach your finger here, and look at My hands; and reach your hand here, and put it into My side. Do not be unbelieving, but believing."

And Thomas answered and said to Him, "My Lord and my God!" Jesus said to him, "Thomas, because you have seen Me, you have believed. Blessed are those who have not seen and yet have believed." And truly Jesus did many other signs in the presence of His disciples, which are not written in this book; but these are written that you may believe that Jesus is the Christ, the Son of God, and that believing you may have life in His name.

When I view this Caravaggio, I sense fear, hurt, anger, loneliness, and gladness. In the biblical passage, fear and gladness are specifically mentioned, and these two emotions seem especially evident in the painting.

The disciples had good reason to fear. Their leader, Jesus, had been executed in a particularly horrific manner. The English word *excruciating* is from the Latin *excruciare*, which is rooted in *cruciare*, meaning "to crucify," signifying pain like that of dying on a cross. Jesus had also been accused of blasphemy before the Sanhedrin—the highest ruling body of the Jews in the first century—and of sedition before the Romans, two capital offenses under each of the respective laws. Such accusations, naturally, led his followers to believe that they might also be targets of the authorities. Otherwise, why did Peter vehemently express denial three times during the Lord's questioning by the high priest?

The Lord's woundedness evokes pain. When people are wounded, physically and emotionally, usually they are guarded. Physicians even describe the appropriate reaction to abdominal palpation in the presence of acute intraabdominal pathology as "guarding," a physiologic response to insult. Such a response is generally an indication of peritonitis, or inflammation of the lining of the abdominal cavity.

In the painting, Jesus is not guarded at all. He is inviting, receptive, encouraging, and almost forceful, as depicted by his left hand gripping Thomas's wrist.[93] It is a perfect metaphor for ultimate vulnerability. Physicians often probe wounds to examine them, drain them of purulence, and irrigate them in an attempt to help them heal. That requires the patients to trust that the physicians know what they are doing, and that they have their patients' best interest at heart. But this trust is the very thing makes patients vulnerable to the physician's probings. Without that trust, anesthesia must be used—which again, requires at least an initial level of trust.

While a physician requires the vulnerability of patients in order to treat them, how trusting are you, as a physician, when it comes to treating your own emotional wounds? How guarded are you? What are you afraid of when it comes to pain? There is a price to pay for having a guarded stance, a protected heart, for disallowing yourself to be vulnerable.

Franciscan priest Richard Rohr, in *Divine Dance*, wrote about vulnerability:

> Did you ever imagine that what we call "vulnerability" might just be the key to ongoing growth? In my experience, healthily vulnerable people use every occasion to

---

93 This is Caravaggio's interpretation of the text. This information is not literally expressed in the biblical passage, though the Lord does invite Thomas to probe, as He says to Thomas, "Reach your finger here ..." (John 20:27).

expand, change, and grow. Yet it is a risky position to live undefended, in a kind of constant openness to the other—because it would mean others could actually wound you (from *vulnus*, "wound"). But only if we choose to take this risk do we also allow the exact opposite possibility: the other might also gift you, free you, and even love you.

But it is a felt risk every time. Every time.[94]

Can you find yourself in the story, in the painting? Are there characters with whom you readily associate? For instance, have you ever felt left out at an important event? Have you ever felt left out by someone important to you?

In my opinion, there can be little doubt that the apostle Thomas had some of those exact same feelings. [95] He had been called and given power by Jesus along with the other apostles. He had expressed courage in persuading the disciples to accompany the Lord back to Jerusalem, even if it meant death.[96] He had been bold in asking where and how to follow the Lord.[97] Yet, in this instance, I imagine he finds himself in the position of being the "last to know." That is where the anger[98] lies in the painting. Thomas had an anger, a passion or deep desire, to know without a shadow of a doubt the veracity of the Lord's bodily resurrection. Because of his passion to know, we know.

Notice the dramatic center of the painting where an obvious arrangement of the heads forms a cross. The focus of attention,

---

94 Richard Rohr, *The Divine Dance* (New Kensington: Whitaker House, 2016), 57.

95 John 20:19–24.

96 John 11:16.

97 John 14:5.

98 Many are uncomfortable with expressing anger in this way. Anger has been conflated with rage. Anger in its purest form is reflective of caring. It informs us of what really matters to us or what has significance. Rage is an impaired expression of fear. See Chip Dodd, *The Voice of the Heart: A Call to Full Living*, 2nd ed. (Nashville: Sage Hill Resources, 2014), 104–105.

however, is not directed toward the center of the image, but to the viewer's left. That is a result of the direction of the subjects' attention along with the direction from which the light is shed on the scene; their attention is focused on the brightest area in this space, to the left of center.

Now examine Thomas's face. There is an intensity to his gaze, perhaps even surprise or astonishment. He is certainly transfixed. Adoration is implied with the kiss he places close to where the imprint of the nail may have been in the Lord's hand. Thomas's posture is also reflective of his total submission.

Consider for a moment the compassion the Lord must have had in His heart for Thomas. Imagine what it took after the three days He had been through: scourging, mocking, desertion, aloneness, abandoned even to a degree by His father as he was left in Hades, the realm of the dead. Yet it appears—both from the text and the masterpiece Caravaggio created—he has only understanding and love for Thomas.

Now imagine yourself in a situation of great duress, perhaps after many difficult days of treating and taking care of patients. Have you ever had a bad day and then taken it out on someone? Maybe you had a complication. Perhaps you carried over your anger, fear, and frustration to the next day and took it out on someone else. Perhaps that person wasn't even involved in the issue that had originally upset you.

As with Champaigne's *Le Christ mort couché sur son linceul*, Caravaggio's *Incredulity of Saint Thomas* also evokes a sense of loneliness, or aloneness—a feeling that comes, in part, from Jesus's aloneness during the events leading up to the encounter with Thomas. In the painting, however, the aloneness is apparent in the positioning and shadowing of Jesus's face. Although He is turned toward the wound, just as the three apostles are, his face is turned in the opposite direction from the faces of the others in the painting.

Loneliness comes all too easily to me. I often don't even notice it, yet I am always immersed in it to a degree. As I mentioned earlier, because I was thirteen years older than my sister—my only sibling—I was, in many respects, psychodynamically an only child. I sat in the back seat of the car alone. I played by myself on vacations. I invented games to stay amused at family gatherings composed only of adults.

Chip Dodd says that loneliness is the feeling we work the hardest to avoid.[99] How many physicians have felt alone and worked harder, longer, and faster, perhaps even accomplishing much professionally only to find themselves bereft of meaningful relationships because they remained guarded? Protecting your heart is understandable. It was completely logical to me—and almost killed me. Living without heart is dangerous.

> *Protecting your heart is understandable. It was completely logical to me—and almost killed me.*

The Bible passage states that the disciples were "glad when they saw the Lord." It makes perfect sense. They thought He was dead, but at that moment He was very much alive and in the flesh, as evidenced by his gaping wounds. The presence of Jesus gave them hope: hope that everything they had been taught and believed was true, hope that the dreams regarding His coming Kingdom were still possible, and hope because their master and teacher was alive. Hopelessness had been dramatically transformed. Jesus showed them His hands and His side. The disciples' experience of gladness immediately follows: "Wherever there is hope there is gladness. Wherever hope is fulfilled there is more gladness."[100] It turns out that we can only be deeply, truly touched if we are open to being known.

---

99   Chip Dodd, *The Voice of the Heart: A Call to Full Living,* 2nd ed. (Nashville: Sage Hill Resources, 2014), 61.

100 Ibid., 135.

If you can give up the right to be on guard with your heart, if you can take the risk of admitting your woundedness, if you can allow yourself to be vulnerable and let others in, you may experience what we all, ultimately, desire: intimacy. Jesus allowed others in, literally to see into Him. Intimacy is "into me see."

That is what is seen in the painting. In a moment of extreme vulnerability, there is the deepest of intimacy. The positioning of Jesus's body allows the viewer into that intimate moment; He is open, even with His wounds. It is a picture of unrelenting, persistent, passionate, forgiving, endless love in spite of our weaknesses, failures, and apparent unworthiness.

That is what I want in life; that is what I believe everyone wants. Yet, for most people, their experiences in this life compel them to believe true intimacy cannot be achieved.

HEALING FROM HURT

Allowing yourself to be vulnerable too often can leave your wounds or woundedness open to exploitation. And when being receptive and open leads to being taken advantage of, you may vow to never let that happen again. But such a vow leaves you refusing to believe the very essence of salvation: you must be willing to suffer hurt in order to experience healing.

> You must be willing to suffer hurt in order to experience healing.

Chip Dodd wrote, "There is mysterious power in the fact that through the pain of hurt, you and I find deeper faith and greater strength."[101] It takes courage to be open and receptive in today's

---

101 Ibid., 54.

world. It takes heart. For too long, I thought life was all about the mind, and that consumed the greater portion of my life.

My understanding was based on an adoption of maladapted Cartesian philosophy in the soul of my being. This in itself is a paradoxical non sequitur. I suspect there was a reason I was so focused on the mind. As many people have, I arrived at a place of hiding from wounds I had carried from my family of origin. Once it is made, a wound is always there. It can be minimized, denied, or camouflaged, but it's always going to leave a mark, a scar.

That's especially true of the wounds that people inflict upon us. Hemingway said, "All people are broken, but some are stronger in the broken places." It's about how people deal with their wounds that matters: some wounds are deadly, some heal and make people stronger. Nevertheless, the wound must be dealt with.

The wound, for most people, was inflicted by a father. I've termed this the *father wound*, as if in doing so, I can distance myself from it. That's the way we tend to deal with such wounds, according to John Eldredge, who wrote, "Our basic approach to life comes down to this: we stay in what we can handle, and steer clear of everything else. We engage where we feel we can or we must—as at work—and we hold back where we feel sure to fail, as in the deep waters of relating to our wife or our children, and in our spirituality."[102]

> *Everyone needs to be initiated into life. Each of us needs someone to show us how to love, how to live, how to engage with our eyes wide open and with our faces to the wind, how to dance in the rain and have heart when all seems lost. It is a Herculean task.*

---

102 John Eldredge, *Fathered by God* (Nashville: Thomas Nelson, 2009), 7.

Although my father was always there for me, I needed more. Every boy and every girl does. I don't believe he had the capacity to provide what I needed. He was fathered by an alcoholic, and even though my father wasn't an alcoholic, some of that rain inevitably flowed downhill. My biggest regret is not what rained upon me, but what I have rained down on my family.

Often, what is needed to heal is to stay vulnerable, to be honest about wounding and woundedness. A spiritual father is often what is needed. To heal simply requires being able to place fingers in His side and to believe that healing is possible.

LIVING WITH YOUR STORY

Healing, therefore, is a form of redemption. To redeem comes from the Latin *redimere*—re- (back) + *emere* (buy)—to buy back. The idea is to regain possession of something in an exchange. Healing comes in response to, or in exchange for, our willingness to acknowledge our hurt to ourselves, to others, and to God. To be open and vulnerable to that admission of hurt allows us to move toward healing. In that process, we recover or redeem a part of ourselves, a part that was wounded. In that sense, it has been redeemed.

Is redemption always possible? What about failures along the way? The truth is that failures are part of the fall, and the fall is part of our story. It is part of your story. What makes me want to behave as though I haven't struggled, stumbled, fallen flat on my face? What is it in me that refuses to embrace my defects, my scars, my wounds, my hurt, and my failures? What makes me love the mountaintop more than the valley?

Stephen, the counselor who first referred me to outpatient treatment, once remarked in a treatment session that his story was much like mine. I told him I was really sorry and thought about how unfortunate he was. He then talked about how much he loved his story. I was baffled. That gnawed at me for several years. I had tremendous difficulty in believing he could love his fall. Understanding that falls are part of the story, and that it's imperative to love that story, was elucidated for me in an unusual way.

One evening, in February 2016, my family was watching the Academy Awards on television when I returned home from a business trip. Brie Larson won the Best Actress Oscar for *Room*, a film about a mother and her five-year-old son who were both imprisoned in a room his entire life. The show included a clip from the film in which Larson, as the mother, described to her son how they both came to be trapped: As a teenager, she was led away by a lie about a dog and then kidnapped. After hearing her tale, the boy shouts, "I want another story!" She snaps back at him, "This is the story you get."

Wow! It hit me like a brick in the forehead. *This is the story I get.* I may loathe the story I have been "given." I may crave another story. But it is my story. I am stuck with it. Much of it seems unfair, but I am responsible *to* my story, and I am responsible for what I choose to do *with* my story. I am learning to love.

The question is, then, are failures God's attempt to lead people to faith? That is difficult to understand. It is tougher to embrace what might be referred to as fallenness or humanness. It is much easier to simply focus on His longsuffering, His love, His mercy and grace. Is the inability to embrace failures a reflection of one's desire to be godlike?

The creation of the universe occurs in Genesis, chapter 1. However, there isn't much story until early in chapter 3, when the fall of man occurs. Falling, then, *is* the story of humanity. We fell in chapter 3 of the first book, and we have stumbled, been pushed down, tripped, thrown ourselves face first to the concrete and laid in our own secretions ever since. There is no redemption without falling, just as there can be no healing without a wound. If you love the redemption, the healing, you must learn to love the fall, the wound. Failing to accept or love your story is a rejection of your woundedness, your humanity, and how you were made.

Physicians are trained to never make mistakes. Side effects and known complications are acceptable, but mistakes are simply unacceptable. *Mistake* can also, in this context, mean that one did not prevent that which is not preventable. I learned that lesson early, while on call as a fresh surgical staff member in the trauma service. I received a page from a nurse, late at night, about an elderly patient who had undergone surgery the previous morning. The patient was under the care of another team. I was simply "covering." I treated her appropriately, but she continued to deteriorate. I called the third-year resident, my immediate superior. I called my chief. They made recommendations. I continued to treat her throughout the night and early morning. It gradually became clear that the elderly woman was in the early process of developing acute renal failure. It was a *fait accompli*.

The next morning, just a few hours later, I was called to see the attending physician in the surgery lounge. I was exhausted, disheveled, and grimy, as my team had worked through the night. He was well-rested, wore a nicely tailored suit, and looked really sharp—even spectacular. He was seated and had me stand before him, where he proceeded—in the most even-tempered, eloquent, and sardonic manner—to question my heritage, my intelligence, and my motivation while underscoring my tremendous capacity for genocide. There was no lecture on the physiology of acute renal failure in the immediate postoperative period, nor was there any suggestion that my training was somehow salvageable. It was humiliating.

Worse, when it was over, I believed he was right. *He's exactly right*, I thought. He merely reinforced what I felt about myself deep down where I dared admit it. I had always felt like a failure, and had worked incessantly to cover it up. But that night I had been discovered. Instead of quitting, however, I resolved to work even harder, to do more, to do better, all while keeping up the charade of my deity perfection.

The patient, by the way, did well and went home a few days later.

During my training, I never forgave myself for mistakes. I collected my failings like notches on a belt. But it also seemed that no one really encouraged any sort of spirit of forgiveness.

In *The Ragamuffin Gospel*, Brennan Manning makes the observation that many moral lapses, failures, and refusals of unmerited favor or grace are not terminal. They are, undoubtedly, the opportunity for painful spiritual growth. They may even be divinely appointed opportunities. Viewed through that lens, sin, repentance, and movement toward God and redemption should be a dance, one in which the second step can only naturally follow the first.

The most beautiful aspect of that viewpoint is the avoidance of toxic shame. Healthy shame recognizes inherent limitations but also strengths or gifts. Toxic shame, on the other hand, continually points to defects and flaws. To be loved requires performance, and when that is not accomplished perfectly, needs cannot be met by anyone. Controlling the environment means self-protection and creating a false self to take care of oneself. That façade is created with the hope that it will be liked, but, instead, it begins to have damaging consequences. The result is that the consequences themselves serve as evidence of the defect, of the flaws, thus proving my original belief:

Through the evidence of these consequences, I believed I was indeed defective. What I had first believed about myself proved to be true.

Speaking your shame takes the power out of it. "It is not unrealistic to presume that later, Peter praised God for the servant girl in Caiphas's courtyard who turned him into a sniveling coward."[103] I believe this idea puts John 21 in a proper context. The Lord essentially speaks Peter's offense out loud in front of his trusted friends. Toxic shame therefore cannot survive. There is no judgment, no denial, no penance. The real gift was to Peter. He subsequently exhibits a humility[104] in Acts not seen in him in the earlier Gospel narratives. Somehow, he was able to forgive himself for the worst kind of treachery: abandonment. He was able to forgive himself for everything. That is a task surprisingly more difficult than it seems.

As I mentioned in chapter 1, "My Fall and Redemption," there is a limbic response to all the ugliness that physicians see every day, and that isn't easily assuaged. It is mediated through the amygdala, and the amygdala never forgets. The feelings associated with the experience can also be just as fresh in the recollection of the event as they were during the event itself. But reconnecting to beauty and truth in the world somehow rights the ship a little bit. As author Madeleine L'Engle wrote, "In art, either as creators or participators, we are helped to remember some of the glorious things we have forgotten, and some of the terrible things we are asked to endure."[105]

I believe we primarily *experience* art. And it is precisely the experience of art that has the capacity to move us. As when we sense the shifting of tectonic plates, seismic rumblings awaken our conscious-

---

103 Brennan Manning, *The Ragamuffin Gospel* (Multnomah Books, 2005), 184.

104 The gift of healthy shame is humility; see Chip Dodd, *The Voice of the Heart: A Call to Full Living,* 2nd ed. (Nashville: Sage Hill Resources, 2014), 120.

105 Madelaine L'Engle, *Walking on Water: Reflections on Faith and Art* (New York: North Point Press, 1980).

ness to our inner emotional life, which for me had been buried as Pompeii had been, beneath a plethora of volcanic ash from earlier explosions. Art speaks to my heart and awakens within me the awareness of a fuller, deeper way of living.

In his memoir, *I'll Run Till the Sun Goes Down*, David Sandum bravely chronicles his battle with depression and his discovery of art. "The powerful world of art had entered my life, with its unspoken language that focused more on feelings than logic. I found many of my emotions buried in the brushstrokes of people who had struggled and painted; Van Gogh, Munch, Kahlo, Cézanne, Kirchner, and Gaugin."[106]

Dr. Heather Stuckey of Pennsylvania State Hershey Medical Center, and Dr. Jeremy Nobel, who holds adjunct appointments at Harvard Medical School and the Harvard School of Public Health, reviewed the current state of research (1995–2007) with respect to art and healing, and found that the majority of studies focused on at least one of four principal types of therapeutic interventions: music, visual art, dance, and/or writing. Their interest was in how these modalities had been used to foster healing and wellness in adults. They concluded that there was ample indication that positive health effects were experienced as a result of engagement with the arts: "The more we understand the relationship between creative expression and healing, the more we will discover the healing power of the arts."[107]

David Sandum, when writing of his experience of art, noted how it touched his soul. His connection to and fascination with art was felt to be out of balance by some of those in his life. Frequent

---

106 David Sandum, *I'll Run Till the Sun Goes Down: A Memoir about Depression and Discovering Art* (Boulder, CO: Sandra Jonas Publishing House, 2015), 99.

107 Heather Stuckey and Jeremy Nobel, "The Connection between Art, Healing, and Public Health: A Review of Current Literature," *American Journal of Public Health* 100, no. 2 (February 2010): 254–263.

arrivals of Amazon packages with books and art DVDs were witnesses of his excess.

I chuckle under my breath and glance up from my MacBook Pro as I type these words to see over a hundred books lying scattered in piles on a large table, which serves as my desk. Thank you, Amazon Prime! I feel as if I am in very good company with those, like Sandum, whose lives are out of balance. At least my life is out of balance with art now. It has been a long journey for a man who was all in his head not that long ago.

FEEL YOUR FEELINGS, TELL THE TRUTH, TRUST THE PROCESS

*There were many things that irritated me about my time in outpatient therapy. That word, **irritated**, is a cover for anger. Words such as **irritation** and **frustration**—which Chip Dodd calls "Christianized anger"—help people remove themselves just a little from their true feelings, which is not always a bad tactic if you are speaking to a coworker or a supervisor, and so on.*

Therapeutic language can be a little scary (read: "fear inducing") to someone who is not used to dealing with emotions and feelings. But when I remove myself from the specific words of those feelings too much, it is easier for me to become unaware of my own feelings, and then difficulties arise. Chip would always say, "Feel your feelings, tell the truth, and trust the process." His instructions seemed too easy to be true—except for two things: 1) They were true; 2) They were anything but easy.

*In therapy, I became acutely aware of how much I lied about how I felt—even to myself. If my apartment mate in therapy asked, "Do you mind if I take a shower first?" I had to examine my answer. Maybe I did mind; maybe I didn't. But to tell my apartment mate that it made me angry that he wanted to be first in the shower every day seemed absurd. Still, by the rules, if I was a little ticked about his going first, I had to use the word **angry**. "Yes, it makes me angry that you want* *to take a shower first every day." It was odd to hear myself verbalize that out loud.*

But then an incredible thing would happen: the world didn't blow up. He might reply, "Oh, okay. No worries. You go first." Or he might say, "I like to go first because if I go last, there is no hot water left and I get angry because your shower was so long."

Either way, those truth-telling interactions really helped us begin to know each other. We were learning to share our inner feelings. Yes, there was a manufactured aspect to it, but I had learned to hide the truth of who I was, even to myself, in order to control my environment. It was very important for me to practice these little things so I could be honest about the bigger things: feelings, those pesky things I could not deal with. I had become very versed at making everyone "okay" at all costs so that no one around me would have feelings. Now, I was learning to live differently.

FIND YOUR
HEART

As you examine your own situation, ask yourself these questions.

▫ What can be the result of a healthy acknowledgment of fear and loneliness?

▫ Learning to love your story is a form of self-compassion. How has it affected you to come to terms with your struggle and even embrace it? Has your struggle to forgive yourself in certain ways affected your ability to forgive others?

▫ What possibilities arise when you allow yourself to be open and vulnerable to hurt?

- Can you think of times in your life when you refused to acknowledge your hurt? If so, what happened as a result?

- What can you offer the world in an undefended stance? What is offered to you in an undefended stance?

SIX

THE GOOD SAMARITAN: THE STORY OF THE OX

The opposite of love is not hate, it is indifference.

—Elie Wiesel

Have you come here for forgiveness? Have you come to raise the dead? Have you come here to play Jesus to the lepers in your head?

—U2

Physicians often find themselves dealing with the proverbial ox in a ditch, a situation with extenuating circumstances that must be considered.[108] Such situations justify bending, or even breaking, the rules. This happened recently when I received a call from an ICU nurse about a twenty-four-year-old man who was dying of metastatic cancer. I was not on call that day, so I vacillated about whether to speak to the nurse or to refer her to my on-call partner. Since the situation was a little unusual—normally, ICU staff would not call me outside the normal rotation—I decided to take the call. I am very glad I did.

---

108 Luke 14:5.

Dennis, the gentleman who was succumbing to metastatic cancer, wanted to go home to die. He wanted to be there with his family, instead of dying in the hospital. For a variety of reasons, his only way to leave the hospital was to submit to a tracheostomy. The family was reluctant to have him undergo the operation unless I could perform the surgery. So, to see him, I delayed ending an already very long day. As it turned out, I had previously cared for all of his children and his wife.

The family expressed their gratitude that I had come, and I was honored that they had so much trust in me. They had originally been told that since I was not on call, I was not obligated to come. But, of course, I was obligated; how could I not be? I am a doctor.

THE PARABLE AND THE PAINTING

Life's interruptions are the subject of one of the best-known biblical narratives—the parable of the Good Samaritan. They are also the subject of Jacopo Bassano's masterpiece, *The Good Samaritan*. The story of the Good Samaritan[109] occurs in the tenth chapter of Luke's Gospel, which has been referred to as the Gospel of the Outcast:

And behold, a certain lawyer stood up and tested Him, saying, "Teacher, what shall I do to inherit eternal life?"

He said to him, "What is written in the law? What is your reading of it?" So he answered and said, "You shall love the Lord your God with all your heart, with all your

---

109 Luke does not, in fact, refer to this story as a parable, though it is commonly referred to as such. Some commentators believe Jesus may be referring to an actual occurrence of which his audience had some knowledge. It is an intriguing consideration; see C. G. Caldwell, *Truth Commentary: Luke* (Bowling Green, Kentucky: Guardian of Truth Foundation, 2011), 631.

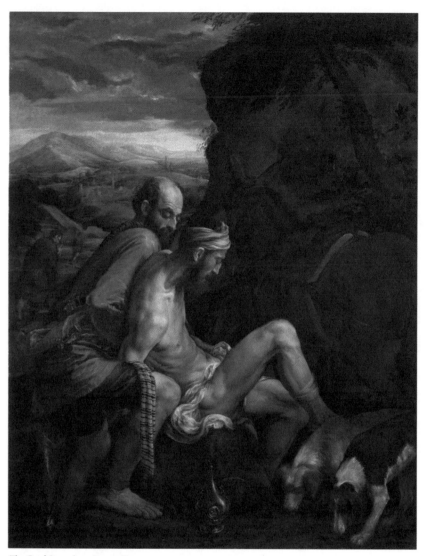

The Good Samaritan, Jacopo Bassano

soul, with all your strength, and with all your mind," and "your neighbor as yourself.'"

And He said to him, "You have answered rightly; do this and you will live."

But he, wanting to justify himself, said to Jesus, "And who is my neighbor?"

Then Jesus answered and said: "A certain man went down from Jerusalem to Jericho, and fell among thieves, who stripped him of his clothing, wounded him, and departed, leaving him half dead. Now by chance a certain priest came down that road. And when he saw him, he passed by on the other side. Likewise a Levite, when he arrived at the place, came and looked, and passed by on the other side. But a certain Samaritan, as he journeyed, came where he was. And when he saw him, he had compassion. So he went to him and bandaged his wounds, pouring on oil and wine; and he set him on his own animal, brought him to an inn, and took care of him. On the next day, when he departed, he took out two denarii, gave them to the innkeeper, and said to him, 'Take care of him; and whatever more you spend, when I come again, I will repay you.' So which of these three do you think was neighbor to him who fell among the thieves?"

And he said, "He who showed mercy on him." Then Jesus said to him, "Go and do likewise."

There is a lot to be gleaned from the events that prompt the telling of the story. The term *lawyer*, used in this New King James Version of the story, is translated in other versions as "an expert in the law" (*nomikos*), which implies someone skilled in interpreting the Jewish scripture and applying the teachings of established rabbis, someone more skilled than the typical scribe. The lawyer asks Jesus for His interpretation of what is necessary to inherit eternal life. Jesus responds by asking the man for his reading of the law. The obvious implication is that the key to eternal life can be found in the law of

God.[110] The expert quotes part of the liturgical shema, Deuteronomy 6:5, and adds Leviticus 19:18, which are referred to in Matthew 22:36–40 as the two greatest commandments.

The lawyer is correct, and the Lord tells him as much. But the lawyer wants to justify himself. I can relate: How many times have I invited a world of trouble by attempting to justify myself? So the lawyer inquires, "Who is my neighbor?" In other words, how far does this thing go? Where can my love end? Who do I get to leave out? What is it going to cost me? The answer in the parable is stunning both in its simplicity and depth.

In viewing Bassano's interpretation of the parable, a sweetness mixed with the joy of gladness envelops me. Serenity exudes from the landscape. The figures of the injured and the one who rescues him from his abject condition are central in the composition.

The victim's downcast gaze suggests his suffering. I imagine him awkward, with somewhat clumsy movements, as he is hoisted onto the waiting horse. His wounds have already been bandaged, as evidenced by the wrapping around his head. The determination of the Samaritan is evident on his face. His entire posture and body position indicate gentle support as he lifts the beleaguered sojourner onto the horse. The flasks of oil and wine are in the foreground, reflective of his care. The Samaritan demonstrates compassion in action. He reveals an anger to try and right the fact that this man has suffered and been left alone.

Only secondarily is attention drawn to the lesser figures behind the Samaritan. Certainly, these figures represent a lost opportunity to have been responsive to the better part of human nature, evoking a

---

110 Tanakh (TaNaKh) is an acronym of the first Hebrew letter of each of the Masoretic text's three divisions: Torah (teaching, aka Pentateuch), Nevi'im (prophets), and Ketuvim (writings, aka hagiographa, or sacred writings).

sense of sadness, fear, and guilt over their actions. The scene causes me to wonder how the priest and the Levite interpreted the Jewish law. Their lack of compassionate response to the scene of suffering creates a sense of loneliness. In Bassano's masterpiece, the Levite is turning away. Though he may have witnessed the assistance being delivered by the Samaritan, it appears he is content to pursue his path of noninvolvement.

When considering that aspect of the painting, anger bubbles up in me, because, as the text notes, the priest and the Levite miss the mark, or fall morally short, through an act of volition. The priest "sees" and the Levite "looks." They didn't inadvertently miss the macabre scene, but instead made a conscious choice to walk away from it. Both pass by on the other side of the road. In that brief description, I detect the notion that neither wanted to get close enough to even feign assistance.

Perhaps the priest and the Levite feared for their own safety. Certainly, steering clear of involvement is safer in many situations. But I am reminded of philosopher Edmund Burke's observation that "the only thing necessary for the triumph of evil is for good men to do nothing."

LIFE HAPPENS

Life is what happens while we are making other plans.[111] I have an agenda nearly every day. I am on a mission to complete it. I may have twenty-five patients to see in the office, fifteen surgeries, a board meeting in Louisville, and a clinic to attend where I see children with special needs. My to-do list might include various phone calls I need to make regarding patient care, getting a coffee with a friend

---

111 Paraphrase of the quotation largely accredited to writer Allen Saunders.

who needs some advice, continuing medical education activities, teaching a Bible class, or giving a lecture. I may be planning a special dinner with my wife. Nothing is inherently wrong with having plans; everyone has them.

However, over time, many people find that the fondest memories are those events that just happened in the interstices of their plans. They are the person you "accidentally" run into, the event that arose without warning.

Some of my family trips have included those memorable interruptions: the snowstorm that cancelled my flight home from Denver a few days before Christmas, the tree that fell and blocked the road as I was coming back from San Antonio, that day our two-car caravan became separated outside Yosemite, Rebecca's bike wreck (while she was on vacation). I have been guilty of stepping over these events in the spaces in and around my plans as if they were cracks in the sidewalk. Slowly, I have learned to be more aware and curious about such apparent intrusions. It may be the person who interrupts me in the operating room, on rounds, or at my favorite coffee shop that brings me the experience I am supposed to have at that very moment. As the noted author C. S. Lewis said, "What one regards as interruptions are precisely one's life." Life's interruptions *are* life. Often, the really important things in our lives aren't the things we plan, they are the things that just happen.

And yet, how common is it to be too busy, too distracted, to notice? How often do people choose to turn away from despair, distress, and suffering? How often do people choose not to get involved out of fear for their own safety or comfort?

NAME YOUR FEAR

Here is one of the most important lessons I've learned through group therapy sessions and as a result of individual counseling: name your fear. What exactly are you afraid of? "Too many of us answer fear by silencing its voice. We run from risk, eliminate trust, hide our dependency, and become fretful and controlling about collaboration."[112]

> *Here is one of the most important lessons I've learned through group therapy sessions and as a result of individual counseling: name your fear.*

Since treatment, I have tried to always move toward fear. It is difficult to do at times. It is a process, and it is progress—not perfection—that matters. The truth is I live with fear. It is the essence of being a doctor. This is a fact that for years I simply did not recognize. I managed my fear by ignoring it, pretending it was nonexistent, as if it could be extinguished through extensive training and repetition coupled with a breadth and depth of knowledge. These things are crucial and they do lessen the fear, but it doesn't eliminate them. Sometimes, in preparation for an operation, I fear on multiple levels. I have a tendency to fear three or four steps ahead, often without recognizing it.

I live with fear because it is the essence of my profession to diagnose, to treat, to manage, to care for, to give recommendations to prevent disease, to control and manage complications, and to prevent unnecessary suffering in those for whom I care. Anticipating problems, pitfalls, potential errors, and misunderstandings is essential. Is it any wonder that many physicians become anxious,

---

112 Chip Dodd, *The Voice of the Heart: A Call to Full Living*, 2nd ed. (Nashville: Sage Hill Resources, 2014), 91–92.

controlling, manipulative automatons? I have jokingly remarked that having obsessive compulsive disorder (OCD) is a great attribute for surgeons. Being obsessive and compulsive makes it a little less likely we will miss some seemingly insignificant detail, which turns out to be critically important. Many a truth is said in jest.

Danielle Ofri discusses her attending duties at New York City's Bellevue Hospital in the book, *What Doctor's Feel: How Emotions Affect the Practice of Medicine.* In a chapter titled "Scared Witless," she writes, "Starting on the wards was always harrowing. It seemed impossible to familiarize myself with every patient, but I had to be sure that I leafed through every chart and at least stopped in at every patient's room for a brief visit, since I was ultimately responsible for every single patient on our ward. Even that minimal amount of attention, though, took hours. I *worried incessantly* (emphasis added) that something would slip under the radar."[113]

The truth is that I ignored, buried, minimized, or talked myself out of all my feelings. I refused sadness, hurt, loneliness, anger, guilt, and shame in addition to fear. There wasn't time to process all of those feelings in real time. There was always the next patient, the next operation, and—let's be honest—I really didn't enjoy all of those feelings, anyway. I am a surgeon.

No one told me that I would worry about patients at night, on vacation, even in the airport. I worry when I lie down and when I wake. I wonder if I have the right diagnosis, if patients have received the correct antibiotic, whether it will even work if they got the right one. I worry about whether or not they will take their medicine, that I explained it correctly or well enough for them to understand. I fear that the operation which removed the malignant tumor, and the

---

113 Danielle Ofri, *What Doctors Feel: How Emotions Affect the Practice of Medicine* (Boston: Beacon Press, 2013), 77.

radiation that follows, may not keep the patient from experiencing a recurrence. I fear that the two-year-old I operated on this morning will bleed following that tonsillectomy. I fear a lot.

Recognizing fear so that you can move into it is imperative in order to gain the wisdom that comes from a healthy appreciation of fear. Ofri used her fear to make sure she did everything possible to ensure her patients received good care. That took collaboration and trust in the team she had around her. We all depend on others—and on God. "The fear of the Lord is the beginning of wisdom."[114]

Recently, I went into a local audio store with my eighteen-year-old son, Caleb, to help him pick out a car stereo for his vehicle. I asked the salesman about the options for Caleb's vehicle, when the stereo could be installed, the details of the warranties, and other buying questions. All the while, Caleb was unusually quiet. Finally, I turned and asked him if he had any questions. He did not. Driving home afterward, I asked him if there was anything he felt we hadn't covered with the salesman. He replied, "Dad, I cannot imagine any exigency that you could possibly have failed to cover."

It made me really sad that my fear about relatively inconsequential things, coupled with my tendency to reside in my mind instead of my heart, had caused me to lose an opportunity to be in a relationship with my son. By being more concerned about the issues surrounding the stereo than I was about *my son's heart*, I had missed an opportunity to truly share the experience with him. Instead, I had managed him and the encounter.

Caleb and I talked about the incident afterward, so in the end everything was fine. He was thankful I was there to help him, and he recognized I had good intentions. And I was fortunate to recognize, in some small way—albeit after the fact—that I had been operating

114 Proverbs 9:10.

out of fear and had lost the opportunity to engage with him. My desire is to be truly *with him* in life. In this instance, it would have been much better if I had noticed the fear in real time and made an adjustment.

When we don't recognize fear for what it is, we have a tendency to exhibit impaired fear or anxiety. Our tendency, then, is to try to hide dependency and become controlling. This does not work well at home, at the office, or in the hospital.

Sometimes this impairment of fear manifests itself as rage. It is a desperate attempt to deny one's heart and avoid pain. "Rage almost always lashes out from deep emotional and spiritual wounds."[115] I believe this is why a lot of physicians rage. I am fairly certain it is why I have raged.

Recognizing and naming your fear can awaken you to the danger, the real danger. It can allow you to admit your limitations and seek collaboration and help. Listening to your fear gives you the opportunity for discernment. If you are unable to name your fear, you are in danger of vacillating between the extremes of cowardly paralysis and arrogant brashness. You become driven by anxiety, or you totally ignore the risks and play the cowboy. Either extreme is fraught with hazard for a physician—and a surgeon, particularly.

Admittedly, I find it remarkably easy to pass by on the other side as the priest and the Levite did. The other side of the road provides the illusion of a lower emotional cost, an easier way to get through the day, to get through life. On the other side, it's easier to get on with a set agenda. The other side allows for the avoidance of people who were probably doing something they should not have done, or were somewhere they should not have been. It allows me to make

---

115 Chip Dodd, *The Voice of the Heart: A Call to Full Living*, 2nd ed. (Nashville: Sage Hill Resources, 2014), 104.

them the problem. Like so many people from all walks of life, I am adept at judging others and justifying myself simultaneously, but in the end, only evil triumphs.

Elie Wiesel, when accepting his Nobel Prize in 1986, said:

> So the question is … when you see someone poor … when you see someone suffering … when you see someone in need. Are you indifferent? Or do you act? The indifference that allowed the world to stand by while the holocaust happened is the same indifference we hear about in the readings today.
>
> The Prophet Amos exclaims: "Woe to us if we are complacent … Woe to us if we are indifferent to those who suffer and are poor." We see this same indifference in the Gospel story of the Rich Man and the Poor Man. The great crime of the Rich man, the sin that would cause him to be forever "tormented" in the eternal flames, was not hate, but indifference.
>
> It was indifference that allowed him to dress in fine linen and purple garments dining sumptuously each day while the poor man named Lazarus laid right there at his doorstep starving and covered with sores. He didn't hate the poor man. He didn't even acknowledge him. He was indifferent.[116]

There is another choice: remaining on the side of the road where the victim lies. It takes heart not to cross over to the other side, to stay on the side of suffering. Being truly present with someone suffering

---

116 Wiesel, Elie, "Excerpts from the Nobel Lecture," Nobelprize.org, December 10, 1986, http://www.nobelprize.org/nobel_prizes/peace/laureates/1986/wiesel-lecture.html.

can be simultaneously the hardest and the easiest thing to do. It is hard to be present on that side of the road because we struggle to find the "right" words to say. We have trouble conveying our feelings in the moment, and many times we don't feel we can do much that is constructive. Yet, it is easy to be present because we don't have to say or do anything but just *be with the victim*. The struggle comes from the uneasiness we feel in the presence of suffering. Walking away from someone in pain makes us feel more comfortable in the moment. While being present can extend the moment of discomfort, it is a way to experience empathic concern or compassion. This experience of compassion has a beneficial effect, not just for the one suffering but also for the one extending it.[117]

Compassion is the recognition of suffering in another and the desire to do something to alleviate it. The Samaritan saw the victim and had compassion. Everything else flows from that recognition of the victim's humanity coupled with the Samaritan's acknowledgment of his own humanity. That it happened in spite of the traditional hatred the Samaritans experienced in Palestine at that time is extraordinary.[118] The oppressed refuses to become the oppressor.

Similarly, it is imperative to find a way to embrace the fullness of your own humanity, to recognize it and have compassion when faced with others' humanity. To truly care for another human means you must also be human.

There is no lack of compassion elicited in the Samaritan when he "sees" the injured man. He uses what he has with him to care for the man's immediate needs, and even places him on his own animal. The

---

117 Adam Grant and Sabine Sonnentag, "Doing Good Buffers against Feeling Bad: Prosocial Impact Compensates for Negative Task and Self-Evaluations," *Organizational Behavior and Human Decision Processes* 111, no. 1 (January 2010), 13–22.

118 John 4:9.

purse with the denarii the Samaritan will use to pay for his patient's recuperation after personally caring for him is on his right hip.

What lengths are you willing to take to serve another? Are you willing to empty your agenda and give your time, resources, expertise, and money to a victim in need? Would you even do that for those who have declared themselves to be your enemy?[119] In Matthew 25, when all the nations are gathered at His throne, what does the text indicate will be the basis of the judgment? Verse 36 further states: "I *was* naked and you clothed Me; I was sick and you visited Me; I was in prison and you came to Me." The passage continues by revealing that those who were blessed to inherit the eternal kingdom didn't even recognize the Lord when they were performing these acts of service. Why? Because when they cared for the least of His brethren, they were actually caring for Him.

It's as renowned author Victor Hugo wrote, "To love another person is to see the face of God." Truly honoring the divine means recognizing the divine that emanates from everyone you meet. We all bear a divine likeness.[120] The Hindu word *namaste* is similar to the Hawaiian word *aloha*, in that it can be both a salutation and a valediction. While *namaste* literally means "I bow to you," it carries with it the connotation that there is a divine spark located in the heart chakra of every person. This gesture reflects an awareness of the divine nature that resides in each human being. Possession of an acute awareness of this fundamental human being-ness does not involve rules, formulas, or what might be termed orthodoxy or religious correctness.

Undoubtedly, the most scathing rebukes from Jesus were levied at the religious elites. He seemed to have little tolerance for those

---

119 Romans 5:5–8.

120 Genesis 1:27.

who only gave pretentious lip service to piety. He even spoke against their efforts at evangelism since they only produced more posers. "You travel over land and sea to win a single convert, and when you have succeeded, you make them twice as much a child of hell as you are."[121]

Still, we all have needs—yes, even physicians. And it's important to recognize our humanity and protect those things that keep us human. "Pretending we don't have needs is playing God—which is not a good position for anyone to be in, not even a healthcare professional."[122]

Perhaps that is why I always feel more like a doctor when I am in impoverished countries. There, I know I am needed and I am free to provide care, using myself as a primary resource. There, I know the patient can sense how much I care. There I find myself unwilling and unable to escape to the far side of the road; there is a "certain man" in the ditch, whichever side I tread. The needs are crushing, and the relief I can offer is always thoroughly appreciated. A couple of vignettes demonstrate what I mean.

A few years back, I was in Honduras on a short mission trip in a remote village outside the capital of Tegucigalpa, which I had been to several times before. We were primarily set up to give out worm medication and vitamins and deal with minor ailments. In reality, we provided more of a public health service than medicine. There was never any doubt, however, about how much the people there appreciated us coming. But a couple of incidents in microcosm reflect part of the struggle of working in places like this.

---

121 Matthew 23:15.

122 Autumn Galbreath, "Physician Burnout," Christian Medical and Dental Associations, *The Point Blog*, May 19, 2016, accessed June 17, 2017, https://cmda.org/resources/publication/physician-burnout.

Late one afternoon, I heard of a young woman whose three-month-old had a fever, but I learned she was planning to wait until the next day to be seen since we were closing up the clinic and getting ready to head back down the mountain. Further questioning revealed that the woman had walked more than two hours to be seen. But on hearing the news that the clinic was closed for the day, incredibly, she calmly turned around and started walking home, stating that she would be back in the morning. Fortunately, one of the locals knew where she lived, so we drove the route until we found her with her child walking along the road. There, alongside the road, I treated the baby's ear infection and gave the mother enough antibiotics and Tylenol for a full course. The next morning, we checked on them both while on our way to the village to open the clinic. The child was afebrile, and looked better overall.

Another morning on that same mission trip, a young man in his early twenties hobbled on crutches into the shack that was my makeshift office. A foul-smelling green drainage exuded from underneath the gauze, and I feared as I unwrapped his injured leg that it was gangrenous. Thankfully, the smell was a folk herbal remedy he had been applying to intact skin.

But the story of his injury was heartbreaking. He had been hit by a car while walking along the main highway ten months prior. He had been taken to a hospital in the city for treatment, where x-rays revealed a tib-fib fracture. He had carried a copy of the film with him to the clinic. Since he had no money, they reduced the fracture, told him to stay off the leg for six weeks, and gave him crutches to use. He had lost his job as a laborer, which was about the only job available in the area for a man of his age. What therefore constituted a relatively minor problem condemned him to a life of even greater destitution.

I could not contain myself. I went out behind the office and sobbed. I have been witness to suffering as a result of poverty in the US, but I have never seen anything like the man I treated that day. In the US, I knew he would have been treated appropriately by someone, somewhere, no matter his ability to pay. I wiped my tears and re-entered the shack. Since I was unable to go with him to the hospital where he would be treated because our team was leaving the country, I called connections there and asked about cost. Then I sent pictures of the fracture to the orthopedic surgeon, and we accounted for any blood or other supplies that might be needed to treat the man. We collected money from the mission team and handed it off to a village authority who agreed to go with the man to the hospital.

In a way similar to the experience of our Lord who was energized by an encounter with another human being at Jacob's well,[123] I am often invigorated when I am at the fountain of living water with a patient. There, in that third-world country, I feel more like a doctor because it's just me and the patient. There are no significant regulations, no demands for time, no administrative relative value units (RVUs), no computer, and no intrusion by the corporate structure.

To be fair, there are challenges to obtaining care for those who need it, particularly since the specialty milieu in which I practice is fairly technologically dependent. I use endoscopes, both rigid and flexible. I operate frequently using a microscope, nerve monitors, a robot, image guidance, and other equipment. They entail a lot of sophistication that takes vigilance, significant cognitive reasoning, and judgment to handle appropriately.

The simplicity of medicine in third-world situations is beautiful, but, if I'm honest, it is to a great degree because there is no intrusion. I am completely free to do the right thing. I may be hindered in

---

123 John 4.

execution. But, if I am, it will be resource driven, and my limitations can be overcome with sacrifice, ingenuity, and—above all—care. I say "care" because when there is simply no way to get something done, for example in Honduras, the patients seem to intuitively know you care. That is what it all boils down to: no one feels uncared

> *That is what it all boils down to: no one feels uncared for, including me. That, to me, is the essence of being a physician.*

for, including me. That, to me, is the essence of being a physician.

I had to travel 2,500 miles, to Honduras, to learn this lesson, but it was well worth it. Compassion is contagious. The more compassion[124] the physician feels, the greater the desire to serve others.

DOCTOR "HERO"

It is clear to me that I want to be the Samaritan. Who doesn't love the hero? However, therein lies an inherent danger, because, in a sense, every young man wants to be a hero.[125] The hero is mythic in American culture, in fictional characters ranging from Aragorn to the Lone Ranger and Spiderman to James Bond.

The role of hero is one that is all too easy to love. When that happens for physicians, the action of the story can then begin to revolve around them, rather than center on the patient, the person whose ultimate good the physician seeks. If physicians see their role as more about being strong, famous, remembered, good, smart, or religious, they risk beginning to serve themselves.

---

124 Compassion can also be referred to as empathic concern. This is in contrast to empathic distress or compassion fatigue.

125 Richard Rohr, *Adam's Return: The Five Promises of Male Initiation* (New York: The Crossroad Publishing Co., 2004), 97.

Therein lies the paradox of Luke's words, "Whoever tries to save his life will lose it, but whoever loses his life will preserve it."[126] The very characteristics that tend to make people good physicians are the very things that make them more susceptible to burnout.[127] It is a haunting irony.

There is also a paradox in the awareness that—though burnout is linked to a personality that has an excessive need for control—it is also associated with a loss of control from a situational standpoint. It is the perfect storm. Recognizing that one is not in total control and is still responsible for the outcome

> *The very characteristics that tend to make people good physicians are the very things that make them more susceptible to burnout.*

anyway, overcompensation seems like a reasonable response. "This need to control everyone and everything, and to refuse to share or delegate power is characteristic of the authoritarian personality type. According to Herbert Freudenberger, the authoritarian individual is especially prone to burnout because of this tendency to do it all, to take on too much, and to overextend him- or herself."[128]

There is a part of me that is glad I had an episode of burnout because it increases the likelihood that I possess the qualities that make a good doctor. Wryly, I call that a sickness. I sincerely believe

---

126 Luke 17:33.

127 Anthony Montgomery, "The Inevitability of Physician Burnout: Implications for Interventions," *Burnout Research* 1, no. 1 (June 2014): 50–56, Science-Direct, accessed June 17, 2017, http://www.sciencedirect.com/science/article/pii/S2213058614000084?via%3Dihub; Troy Parks, "What Makes Doctors Great also Drives Burnout; A Double-Edged Sword," AMA Wire, June 21, 2016, accessed June 17, 2017, https://wire.ama-assn.org/life-career/what-makes-doctors-great-also-drives-burnout-double-edged-sword.

128 C. Maslach, *Burnout: The Cost of Caring* (Los Altos, CA: Malor Books, 2003), 113.

that my early desire to be a physician came from the purest and most genuine of places. It arose as an untainted desire from my true self.

But that desire in the midst of daily life can lead those with the best intentions into dangerous terrain where it insidiously draws them into denying their humanity. Most often this condition manifests itself in long periods of sleep deprivation, or in failure to take a vacation or time off, or when people work inordinately as if everything were solely dependent on them. What begins as a favor can become an erased boundary. For example, you may find yourself *always* being available to patients whether by text, messaging, or cell phone—operating every Saturday without making a conscious decision to do so, never being able to say no to a request, no matter how absurd or intrusive.

It is a difficult tightrope physicians walk: the more compassionate they are, the greater their desire to serve others. Without understanding the need for balance, physicians end up drawing continually from a well of resiliency that may run dry. Being able to give assistance to the man in the ditch and to remember the purpose, the calling, may just help the well to never dry up.

I find it compelling to think of the Good Samaritan as a story. He undoubtedly had a lifetime full of plans, but the thing for which he has been remembered for some two thousand years is the compassion he demonstrated when he was on his way somewhere else. Life interrupted his plans and he took the time to care.

CARING FOR THE COMPASSIONATE

We all know physicians who are so consumed with fear that they trust no one and nothing. They are those physicians who double-check schedules, brood over the smallest decisions, rarely relinquish any amount of control, suspect everyone of attempting to thwart their efforts, and erupt at the slightest hint of a mistake or error on the part of others. Perhaps this describes you.

The sad part of this equation is that these doctors are usually harder on themselves than they are on others. It is the constant threat and fear of failure that forces them to reach for and attempt to control things that are beyond their ability to control. While this is an effort to manage their anxiety, ultimately it is a feeble attempt at independence and sovereignty that only increases the anxiety. "In order to control anxiety we focus on preventing rejection, humiliation, failure, not being acknowledged for our achievements, not performing to someone else's standard, not being loved and all the things in the future we cannot touch."[129]

Naming your fears, being aware of them—even moving into them—brings you into relationship with your heart, which is why it takes courage to do it. It brings you to an awareness of your limitations and your neediness. You can know yourself and then have yourself to give to others. If you are not in possession of yourself, you have nothing to give.

Fortunately, compassion can be taught.[130] The first step is to be compassionate to yourself. "The secret to caring for the patient is caring for oneself, while caring for the patient."[131] When in touch with your own emotions (having you), you can effectively empathize and have compassion for another (giving yourself to others).

Compassion must become a river that flows upstream and downstream. Medical care in the United States needs to blow the dams and stop interrupting the natural flow of compassion between humans who come together to share a healing experience. "Com-

---

129 Chip Dodd, *The Voice of the Heart: A Call to Full Living*, 2nd ed. (Nashville: Sage Hill Resources, 2014), 100–101.

130 Susanne Leiberg, Olga Klimecki, and Tania Singer, "Short-Term Compassion Training Increases Prosocial Behavior in a Newly Developed Prosocial Game," *PLoS One* 6, no. 3 (March 9, 2011): e17798, https://doi.org/10.1371/journal.pone.0017798.

131 Lucy Candib, *Medicine and the Family: A Feminist Perspective* (New York: Basic Books, 1995), 230.

passion is a universal human experience in response to suffering. Organizations can very effectively extinguish it. "[132]

FIND YOUR
HEART

As you examine your own situation, ask yourself these questions:

- How do we train physicians so they have a better chance of staying human through the process, so that they mitigate burnout or are equipped to avoid it altogether?

- What did your medical school/training program do well in this regard? Where do you feel it fell short or could have done better?

- What about your current situation? Hospital? Practice Organization?

- What would you like to change about yourself? Would you like your life to be different?

- When did you feel most alive during the past six months? What were you doing? How did it happen and what was it that allowed you to feel life to that extent?

Consider this exercise to help you on your own healing journey:

- List ways in which you have misused your self-will to control other people or things.

---

132 Beth Lown, "Activating Compassion: Implementing a Framework for Compassionate, Collaborative Healthcare" (keynote presentation at Harvard Medical School "Compassion in Practice" course, October 28–29, 2016).

SEVEN

THE RETURN OF THE PRODIGAL SON

*You must believe in truth that whatever God
gives or permits is for your salvation.*

—Catherine of Siena

Forgiveness is the giving, and so the receiving, of life.

—George MacDonald

Rembrandt's masterpiece, which hangs in Catherine the Great's Hermitage in St. Petersburg, Russia, was the nascent though indirect impetus for this book. I was visiting the meeting of the West Virginia State Medical Association at the Greenbrier resort and rereading Nouwen's inspirational memoir, *The Return of the Prodigal Son: A Story of Homecoming*, when I was touched by his story about being spiritually moved by a piece of classical art. It reminded me of my encounter with the works of Murillo, Honthorst, Bassano, and Caravaggio in London several years prior.

The nudge to write came early on a Sunday morning. It had been about fifteen months since my time at the CPE, and the world of feelings was still opening new experiences for me in the outer world through a growing awareness of my inner one.

The idea came in a manner I can only describe as an epiphany. Evelyn and I had wanted to browse some of the shops on the Greenbrier property, but the store where we had intended to spend the majority of our time was closed. Instead, we wandered into one of the other retail stores just after I told her of the idea that had come to me that morning: I would write a book in which classical art played a major role. When we entered the shop and began to look around, the owner asked if we were Christians. It was a good bet because Evelyn was looking at pendant crosses.

The owner then produced a well-worn *Strong's Exhaustive Concordance of the Bible* with tattered pages bound by duct tape. It was without a doubt one of the most well-read books I have ever seen. She gleefully removed a large manila envelope from within its pages and pulled out a number of classical Renaissance art prints. "I just got these in yesterday," she said. I have been waiting to show them to someone." Evelyn and I looked at one another in shared astonishment. The owner showed us the prints.

I remember feeling glad, but with some fear and shame. It was a very affirming experience. I set my heart to write that morning.

THE PAINTING

Arguably, *The Return of the Prodigal Son* by Rembrandt Harmenszoon van Rijn is one of the last, most popular, and best-known works of the Dutch Golden Age master. The passage Rembrandt portrays in this painting is in Luke 15:11–32:

> A certain man had two sons. And the younger of them
> said to his father, "Father, give me the portion of goods

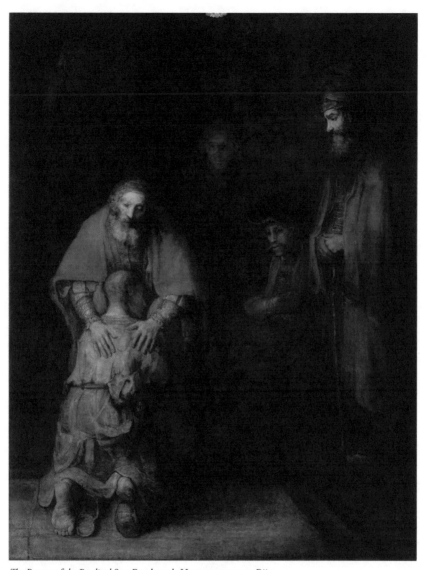

The Return of the Prodigal Son, Rembrandt Harmenszoon van Rijn

that falls to me." So he divided to them his livelihood. And not many days after, the younger son gathered all together, journeyed to a far country, and there wasted his possessions with prodigal living. But when he had spent all, there arose a severe famine in that land, and he began to be in want. Then he went and joined himself to a citizen of that country, and he sent him into his fields to feed swine. And he would gladly have filled his stomach with the pods that the swine ate, and no one gave him anything.

But when he came to himself, he said, "How many of my father's hired servants have bread enough and to spare, and I perish with hunger! I will arise and go to my father, and will say to him, 'Father, I have sinned against heaven and before you, and I am no longer worthy to be called your son. Make me like one of your hired servants.'"

And he arose and came to his father. But when he was still a great way off, his father saw him and had compassion, and ran and fell on his neck and kissed him. And the son said to him, "Father, I have sinned against heaven and in your sight, and am no longer worthy to be called your son."

But the father said to his servants, "Bring out the best robe and put it on him, and put a ring on his hand and sandals on his feet. And bring the fatted calf here and kill it, and let us eat and be merry; for this my son was dead and is alive again; he was lost and is found." And they began to be merry.

Now his older son was in the field. And as he came and drew near to the house, he heard music and dancing. So he called one of the servants and asked what these things meant. And he said to him, "Your brother has come, and because he has received him safe and sound, your father has killed the fatted calf."

But he was angry and would not go in. Therefore his father came out and pleaded with him. So he answered and said to his father, "Lo, these many years I have been serving you; I never transgressed your commandment at any time; and yet you never gave me a young goat, that I might make merry with my friends. But as soon as this son of yours came, who has devoured your livelihood with harlots, you killed the fatted calf for him."

And he said to him, "Son, you are always with me, and all that I have is yours. It was right that we should make merry and be glad, for your brother was dead and is alive again, and was lost and is found."

Luke 15 is commonly referred to as the chapter of lost things: the sheep (verses 3–7), the coin (verses 8–10), and the son. The contrast in attitudes and societal positions among our Lord's audience in this passage is striking. The publicans and sinners draw near to hear while the scribes and Pharisees murmur about His associations (verses 1–2). It is these attitudes that frame the parables in this chapter.

Coming full circle in a healing journey is about remembering how it felt at the beginning of the journey. For me, that's about recognizing the younger son in myself, rejecting everything that I was raised to do or thought I wanted in terms of the humanity of it. I went away to a foreign country and lost my heart, and then I came home to find it. I can still be a doctor and have my heart, and in fact be a better doctor with my heart, but it requires that I, in a sense, fully live the paintings that I've discussed in this book: stand before the accuser, suffer well, accept my position and admit my helplessness, recognize my own mortality, be open to my wounds. I must be willing to take time out of my day to be the Samaritan but not demand to be the hero.

THE YOUNGER SON

The emphasis both in the passage and in the painting is on the return. In the son's return, there is undeniable deep gladness. The eyes are drawn to the father's embrace of his son to the left of center. His expression and the placement of his hands are unmistakably the gentle embrace of understanding, loving compassion. That aspect of the scene dominates the painting.

An earnest sadness also envelops me when I look at the painting, sadness at what the younger son and the father have suffered. The experiences that brought them to this moment speak of what each has lost in their separate, but intertwined journeys.

I also sense hurt. Hurt, I have learned, is about expressing the need for healing. That requires an admission of hurt, or an admission of the fact that we have hurt others. "Vulnerability to hurt initiates a balm for your pain."[133] In the painting, the son expresses his vulnerability through his hurt and in seeking the forgiveness of his father. "I have a wound that needs healing," he says. Standing, recently, at the foot of this magnificent painting at the Hermitage, I felt all the hurt of my own wandering and heartless living envelop me.

Without the admission of hurt, the prodigal son does not return and is therefore not able to receive the privilege of experiencing his father's forgiveness. Without the admission of my own hurt, I also stay in that heartless foreign land. That is the value of feeling your own hurt: in doing so, you can experience the gift of healing.[134]

---

133 Chip Dodd, *The Voice of the Heart: A Call to Full Living*, 2nd ed. (Nashville: Sage Hill Resources, 2014), 53.

134 Ibid.

But there can be no return, no homecoming, without there first being a "leaving." In that home-leaving, there is an implicit rejection of home, how we were made, who we are, and often all of these at once. It is a tragedy.

In that rejection, I recognize the younger son in myself. Nearly everyone leaves home and has to journey back. As I said previously, we all have a homecoming we seek. That journey is known as healing, recovery, deliverance, absolution, redemption, salvation, and forgiveness. It is experienced, finally, most succinctly, as love.

The prodigal son, in leaving, takes the inheritance that legitimately would be his only upon his father's death. Nouwen indicates that his request to be given his inheritance reflects his impatience in waiting for his father's death.[135] It would be like saying, "Dad, I wish you were dead." In that whole process of leaving and rejecting the father, there is a profound hurt and sadness.

That would be insult enough. But then the son spends the inheritance in prodigal living, or wasteful, lavish spending, which is undoubtedly in opposition to everything he was taught in his father's house and his own country. Seeking approval and affirmation from people and in places that takes the heart far away from home is comparable to blowing an inheritance. Seeking approval comes from an inherent sense of worthlessness. Part of the son's problem is he thinks too little of himself. How many times have I have left home and blown it out of a sense of inner emptiness? Too often.

Leaving home in a spiritual sense is not just leaving God—it is leaving self. These two "leavings" are, in a sense, synonymous. What does God want from any of us anyway? He doesn't need anything we have. He wants a relationship with us; he wants us to walk with

---

135 Henri Nouwen, *The Return of the Prodigal Son: A Story of Homecoming* (New York: Doubleday, 1992), 35.

Him[136] and know Him.[137] All we can give to God, ultimately, is what He gave us in our beginning, which is our true self.[138]

The prodigal son loses his true self in the far country. It could be argued that he lost his true self before he left home, and then proved that when he left physically. He only comes to his senses when he loses everything, including his dignity. He hits bottom. Caring for swine, as a Jew, alone and feeling the desire to eat from the pig's trough, he remembers that he is his father's son; he remembers who he is. Then, as the text reads, "He came to himself," and, thus, he comes to an awareness of his true self. It is as if he awakens from a nightmare of his own creation.

Avoiding a world of hurt, guilt, and shame comes from remembering who you are, or more accurately, rediscovering who you are. As Saint Teresa of Avila wrote in *Interior Castle*, "For the most part all of these trials and disturbances come from our not knowing ourselves."[139] Many people never manage to begin the search for their true self.

The Cistercian monk Thomas Merton said, "For me to be a saint means to be myself. Therefore the problem of sanctity and salvation is in fact the problem of finding out who I am and of discovering my true self."[140] That is radical thinking for establishment religion because it feels uncontrollable—and it is. It is lamentable that religion has attempted to substitute the "keeping of rules" for transformative experiences or true conversions.

---

136 Micah 6:8.

137 John 17:3.

138 Thomas Merton, *New Seeds of Contemplation* (New York: New Directions Publishing, 1961), 31.

139 Teresa of Avila, *Interior Castle*, IV: 1, 9.

140 Thomas Merton, *New Seeds of Contemplation* (New York: New Directions Publishing, 1961), 31.

Augustine of Hippo said, "God is more intimate to me than I am to myself." Getting a sense of God's immanence, His presence in and around you, can change how you relate to everything. Sensing His presence can allow you to stay more present. There is a "fundamental oneness and wholeness in God where our desire and God's desire are the same ... Wholeness is our birthright. Oneness is our most original state of being."[141] The merging of your own desire with God's desire is a result of finding your true self fashioned after him. There isn't anything to fear in that, other than the loss of the ego.[142]

What is it about humans that we have to hit absolute bottom, lose nearly everything, including our "self," before we become willing? We must be forced to give up our programs for "happiness at last," it seems. In every moment, but particularly when a person is suffering, it is important to ask, where is God and what is He up to? That was one of the questions plaguing Habakkukk when he saw the spiritual condition of the people of Judah.[143] He had even more questions when he was informed that God's answer to the moral depravity he witnessed was that the Chaldeans would come as conquerors.[144]

Something counterintuitive is at work here. The difficulty arises with the misuse or abuse of will, instead of bringing it into agreement with God's intention. The more dependent on God you become, the more independent you in fact are. Step three of the AA twelve steps states, "Made a decision to turn our will and our lives over to the care of God as we understood Him."[145] When you bring your will into

---

141 Chuck DeGroat, *Wholeheartedness: Busyness, Exhaustion and Healing the Divided Self* (Grand Rapids, Michigan: William B, Eerdmans Publishing Company, 2016).

142 While loss of the ego is not to be feared, it is often described as a type of death.

143 Habakkuk 1:2–4.

144 Ibid., 5–14.

145 W. Bill, *Twelve Steps and Twelve Traditions* (Alcoholics Anonymous World Services, 1981), 35.

alignment with His will, you begin to use it appropriately. Recognizing your place—that is true humility.

The AA program also teaches that "so long as we were convinced that we could live exclusively by our own individual strength and intelligence, for just that long was a working faith in a Higher Power impossible."[146] But, as Richard Rohr writes, "How can we surrender unless we believe there is someone out there trustworthy to surrender to?"[147] Yet, how can that level of surrender be accomplished without some sort of metaphysical mooring?

Notice how the prodigal son practices what he plans to tell his father (verses 18–19). What makes a person rehearse a speech that is never going to be given? Why do we often feel explanations are necessary? Get defensive so quickly? Isn't it the way we treat each other as humans? Our life experiences, then, affect how we perceive the heart of God.

I thus have the very human tendency to believe that all love is conditional, that love is performance based. That is not, however, how He treats us. Since we are not accustomed to such a deeply generous, magnificent, welcoming love, we hesitate to believe it can be true. We have all been burned before. Disbelief in His love is based on our worldly experience. How much of your vision of God is tainted by how you have been treated?

There can be significant intransigence among peers when you decide to admit your weakness and get help. It is sometimes hard to leave the "far country" because the citizens of that country want to keep you there, wallowing in the mire, while others "at home" don't exactly welcome your return. As did the elder son in the parable,

---

146 Ibid., 72.

147 Richard Rohr, *Everything Belongs: The Gift of Contemplative Prayer* (New York: The Crossroad Publishing Co.), 69.

those "at home" conclude you "blew it" and you deserve to suffer all the consequences.

THE ELDER SON

When it became obvious that I needed to take some time off, I approached my partners with open vulnerability about what was going on, and why. I divulged my diagnosis of PTSD-associated depression, and committed to making up any missed calls. Still, I acknowledged that they would have to care for some of my patients who needed treatment or follow-up in the coming weeks. I was very appreciative I had partners.

I had been on the KMA Board of Trustees for over ten years, and, during that time, I heard regular reports from the Kentucky Board of Medical Licensure (KBML). I knew, as a result of that experience, that my colleagues might have some concerns that I was attempting to hide a drug or alcohol problem. So I asked if they had questions or concerns about why I was leaving, and I acknowledged that my leaving was unusual. For example, I had never heard of anyone taking time off like this without being forced to do so. But I told them that was exactly what I was doing; I was taking time off to get help before I had a bigger problem.

I related that the regulations in Kentucky were such that even if I self-reported to the KBML and voluntarily went to rehab for a drug or alcohol problem, I would have to be there for three months. So the length of my treatment period alone (six weeks) should give them assurance that I was being transparent. I invited them to call the board of licensure if they had any doubts and check the regulations for themselves. No one checked. Instead, they wished me well.

One of my partners even related that he had been in therapy himself after his parents' divorce and he supported me fully.

When I returned to resume practicing six weeks later, I found that the same partner who had been in therapy had filed a letter of inquiry with the credentials committee of one of the hospitals where I held privileges. That made it necessary for me to defend myself before the chairman of that committee. I also held credentials at another outpatient facility that had come up for renewal in routine fashion. As was customary, our group had always filled out recommendations for each other. One of the forms had a space to note any problems that would keep me from practicing and asked whether I had been treated for alcohol or drug abuse. My partner had written in that space that I had gone away for six weeks and he had "no idea why," which left me with more explaining to do.

In a way, I think it was good for me to have to admit to other colleagues what happened and why. But I don't believe my partner's comment was given with good intentions. He wanted to damage me—and it did hurt me deeply. I was reminded of the words of Joseph at the end of Genesis. His brothers sold him into slavery, but he advanced to the right hand of Pharaoh. When his brothers feared reprisal, he said, "But as for you, you meant evil against me; *but* God meant it for good."[148] Although I experienced anger about how I was treated by some physicians, fortunately for my recovery those unsupportive associates voluntarily left town over the ensuing year or two for unrelated reasons. Even though coming home is not always easy, is not always well received and can be a challenge, the journey is still worth the trip.

In Rembrandt's painting, the elder son is in the company of three onlookers. In some representations of the masterpiece it can

---

148 Gen. 50:20.

be difficult to see the figure in the doorway over the father's right shoulder. Rembrandt took artistic liberty with the depiction of the parable since the elder son does not actually witness the reunion of his father with the prodigal son. Each of the impassioned onlookers appearing in the scene is dramatically removed by a combination of distance and shadowing, with the distance creating a sense of tension, particularly between the elder son and the embrace he witnesses. It is difficult for me to admit the anger I feel when I consider the elder son. My anger is, in part, a reflection of the anger the elder son projects onto the parable; he is pictured above the father and his brother, and is looking down his nose at them. He also is in a very real sense as lost as the younger son; he just lost himself without leaving home.

The elder son feels the father loves him less, even though the father runs to greet the elder son as he did the younger: "He lovingly addressed the son in the dearest of terms: *teknon*, child."[149] I missed that part of the parable initially because of my anger toward the elder son. The elder son's words are self-pitying, self-righteous, jealous words. They are words from a heart that feels it has never received what it was due.

Yes, I am the elder son in my family, but I have also played the elder son in life. I have been smug, self-righteous, aloof, removed, and accusatory. Similarly, many people do not feel appreciated or honored while others they deem less worthy receive more attention. Those expectations are often a person's own undoing.

In spite of the accusations made against the heart of his father, in the parable the father invites the elder son to the celebration. Will he come? That part of the story in the parable is left untold. The deeper

---

149 C. G. Caldwell, *Truth Commentary: Luke* (Bowling Green, Kentucky: Guardian of Truth Foundation, 2011), 855.

question is, will those who play the elder son in life, when invited, come—to the joy of the Father?

THE FATHER

While I have also been the elder son, as the father of a daughter and two sons, I also understand the father's heart. However, the courage and the heart that the father demonstrates, arising from the profundity of his love, is nearly unfathomable to me. Despite the unreasonable demands of the younger son—the implicit accusations, the rejection of the father's way of life and his care, and ultimately, of the father himself—the father gives the son what he desires and lets him go. The father surely knows the pain to come, the heartache to be suffered, the war to be waged, and yet he doesn't scream, yell, plead, or cajole. "It is precisely the immensity of divine love that is the source of the divine suffering."[150]

Upon the prodigal son's return, the father runs to greet him. In Rembrandt's masterpiece, even the posture with which the father receives the prodigal son is indicative of his receptiveness: the position of the father's hands, the tilt of his head, the roundness of his shoulders, his gaze. The text reads, "He saw him afar off." Expectantly watching, the father has anticipated the prodigal's return and cannot contain his joy to hold him again when he sees him. The father's love, a reflection of divine love, offers the freedom to reject love or to love in return.

The concept Rembrandt captures in that embrace summarizes well the biblical passage stylistically. That concept could change everything if I were to accept it in the core of my being. Is this not

---

150 Henri Nouwen, *The Return of the Prodigal Son: A Story of Homecoming* (New York: Doubleday, 1992), 95.

the God we all want to believe in, one who can only find blessing in his heart? How many of my struggles would dissipate if I could let the truth of God's non-comparing love permeate my heart?

Do I believe I am worth finding? There is a promise intimated by the Father's son in the Sermon on the Mount:

> Ask, and it will be given to you; seek, and you will find; knock, and it will be opened to you. For everyone who asks receives, and he who seeks finds, and to him who knocks it will be opened. Or what man is there among you who, if his son asks for bread, will give him a stone? Or if he asks for a fish, will he give him a serpent? If you then, being evil, know how to give good gifts to your children, how much more will your Father who is in heaven give good things to those who ask Him! Therefore, whatever you want men to do to you, do also to them, for this is the Law and the Prophets.[151]

The request is for relationship. The promise is of self-emptying love. That is the accusation the elder son brings against the father. Essentially, he says, "How dare you be so extravagantly wasteful with your love?" His charge against the father is that of prodigal loving.

God wants a relationship with us and invites us into that divine dance, asking only that we reflect the love we so desperately desire and He so richly lavishes upon us into the world. It is a world that could use it.

The elder son's charge against the father is that of prodigal loving.

---

151 Matthew 7:7–12.

GENUINELY HAPPY AT LAST

One day, in the last few weeks of therapy, I was walking through a local grocery store and I realized that I was truly, genuinely happy. That gladness was genuine because it was rooted in a recognition that I had begun to accept who I was and how I was made. In the midst of experiencing that gladness, I also realized some sadness and shame because I had been, and was, in need of recovery. There was also some sadness and anger over the fact that my recovery had not come earlier in life. I detected some fear that, without continued effort, I was in danger of a relapse.

I was working through my feelings—fear, anger, shame, sadness, and gladness—while walking down the aisles picking up items for dinner for the guys back at the apartments. Then, suddenly, it registered: without the ability to feel the fear, anger, shame, and sadness, I would be incapable of feeling glad.

*The joy of that moment was so huge that it helped me appreciate what a gift the ability to feel was. In order to feel gladness, I must be willing to feel **all** of the feelings. I had always run from the experiences of loneliness, fear, shame, sadness, anger, and hurt; in doing so, I had unwittingly robbed myself of joy. More importantly, I had robbed myself of living. Denying my heart had, eventually, resulted in the depression that drove me to seek help.*

Fortunately, I awakened in the pig's sty and possessed the insight (with help) to trust the heart of the Father. He had seen me from afar, and I was resting in his embrace.

FIND YOUR
HEART

As you examine your own situation, ask yourself these questions:

- How have you treated life more as a destination than a process? How has this helped or harmed your progress?

- How has your experience of life affected your perception of the character or heart of the Father?

- In what ways have you played the role of the elder son in your life? How has that kept you from celebrating others? How has it kept you from a deeper experience of life?

- Thomas Merton said, "The biggest human temptation is to settle for too little."

- In what ways have you settled for too little and how has that affected you? What would it look like if you were to "stop settling?" Think about that possibility. How does it make you feel?

How we train and educate physicians can help to reduce the causes of stress and assist doctors in increasing their capacity for the development of resilience. Increasing stress and reduced resilience tends to lead to burnout.

Individuals need their own program to combat burnout, not because it is necessarily their fault. Individuals are not responsible for their burnout, but they are responsible to it. They are responsible to the malady, not for it. Consider living the paintings discussed in this book to help you find your heart and its voice:

- Stand before the accuser and suffer well.

- Admit helplessness.

- ❑ Recognize your mortality.

- ❑ Be open to your wounds.

- ❑ Serve others selflessly.

- ❑ Rest in the joyful embrace of a prodigal God.

EIGHT

SEE BEAUTY AND REVIVE THE HEART

What is to give light must endure burning.

—**Viktor Frankl**

I made it into and through medical school and a residency in large part by lowering my head, keeping my eye on the goal, and plowing ahead no matter what. I have stories to tell that reflect the absurdity of the life I lived. All doctors have such stories.

When I was in treatment at the CPE, Chip Dodd shocked me one day by comparing physicians to Navy SEALS. As a group, he said, physicians are every bit as tough as the elite fighting force. Physicians can take anything and keep on working, he said. We were trained to do that, to ignore all discomfort.

Having been in uniform as a reservist, and on active duty in the medical corps for a short period of time in Operation Desert Storm and Desert Shield, I was reluctant to validate his comparison. That's partly because I hold the men and women of the armed services in very high esteem for their sacrifices and service to the country, especially those who are in elite units such as the Navy SEALS.[152]

---

152 Most of the time, physicians do not serve in military theaters of operation where people are trying to kill us. ER doctors in inner city hospitals might be an

When he began to describe in detail how physicians function, however, I began to grant some credence to his point. He said that we deny normal bodily functions as well as family and human demands in order to accomplish missions. That much is true. While performing surgery, I have gone eight to fourteen hours without a break for food, water, or bathroom relief too many times to count. I have slept less than eight hours in one week, and have consequently fallen asleep while standing and writing orders in an ICU. I have been called away on a moment's notice for work and have answered those last-minute calls no matter what is going on in my personal life. I have very high personal standards of performance, and I expect the same of my colleagues. In my mind, I must keep working and serving no matter what. My training has taught me well.

What is interesting is that is the demands placed on me are not particularly exceptional. In fact, as an otolaryngologist, the absurd demands placed on me are probably lower in intensity than the demands placed on many of my peers. We have all learned how to put all of our feelings, needs, longings, and desires on hold, until such time as they may be worked into the schedule. Perhaps I learned too well.

Emotional exhaustion, depersonalization, and a low sense of personal accomplishment or burnout[153] are responses so common in medicine that physicians have begun to consider the appropriate steps to combat what is approaching a pandemic. According to the *Medscape Otolaryngologist Lifestyle Report 2017*, more than half of otolaryngologists (53 percent) are burned out, which is slightly above the overall rate for all physicians. [154]

---

exception.

153 C. Maslach, *Burnout: The Cost of Caring* (Los Altos, CA: Malor Books, 2003), 2.

154 Carol Peckham, "*Medscape Otolaryngologist Lifestyle Report 2017: Race and Ethnicity, Bias and Burnout*," Medscape, January 11, 2017, accessed April

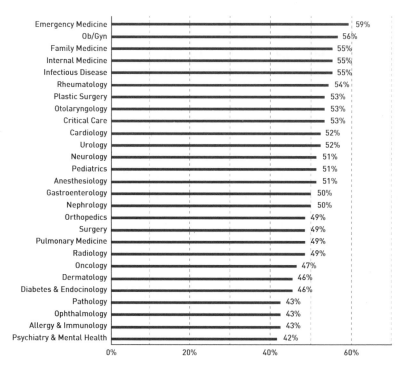

WHICH PHYSICIANS ARE MOST BURNED OUT?

Specialty	Burnout Rate
Emergency Medicine	59%
Ob/Gyn	56%
Family Medicine	55%
Internal Medicine	55%
Infectious Disease	55%
Rheumatology	54%
Plastic Surgery	53%
Otolaryngology	53%
Critical Care	53%
Cardiology	52%
Urology	52%
Neurology	51%
Pediatrics	51%
Anesthesiology	51%
Gastroenterology	50%
Nephrology	50%
Orthopedics	49%
Surgery	49%
Pulmonary Medicine	49%
Radiology	49%
Oncology	47%
Dermatology	46%
Diabetes & Endocinology	46%
Pathology	43%
Ophthalmology	43%
Allergy & Immunology	43%
Psychiatry & Mental Health	42%

Figure 8-1. *The overall burnout rate is 51 percent, a more than 25 percent increase over just four years.*[155]

Noted physician Starla Fitch in her book *Remedy for Burnout: 7 Prescriptions Doctors Use to Find Meaning in Medicine,* is prescriptive in her recommendations to prevent and treat burnout: the development of resilience, the practice of faith, the cultivation of feelings of self-worth, the practice of creativity, employment of compassion, development of compassion, and encouraging connection.[156]

Dike Drummond, a Mayo-trained family physician and burnout specialist, argues for a different paradigm. He identifies burnout as a

---

29, 2017, http://www.medscape.com/features/slideshow/lifestyle/2017/
otolaryngology#page=2.

155 Ibid.

156 Starla Fitch, *Remedy for Burnout* (Minneapolis: Langdon Street Press, 2014).

dilemma, not a "problem." Burnout is not something to be prevented as much as it is something to be handled or dealt with appropriately.[157] He categorized the recommendations to treat the dilemma of burnout as tools that decrease stress, help recharge an individual, and pursue similar goals on an organizational basis.[158] In a meta-analysis published in *Lancet*, Colin West, Liselotte Dyrbye, Patricia Erwin and Tait Shanafelt identified 2,617 articles of which fifty-two met inclusion criteria. These data indicate meaningful reductions in physician burnout can be achieved through both individual-focused and organizational strategies.[159] We need to implement both individual and organizational strategies.

However, that having been delineated, I believe that physicians need to take responsibility for their own well-being. The organization you work in may not *care* as the institutions that have instituted structural change would. Or your organization may be so listless and unresponsive that depending on its leaders to change the culture—or suggesting that a change is needed—would be unrealistic and unwise. You may be stuck with your organization or institution for a variety of reasons that are beyond your reasonable control. "When we are no longer able to change a situation, we are challenged to change ourselves," Austrian neurologist, psychiatrist, and Holocaust survivor Viktor Frankl wrote.[160]

I am not arguing that you can insulate yourself from any chance of burnout in any situation. There are environments where almost all

---

157 Dike Drummond, *Stop Physician Burnout: What to Do When Working Harder Isn't Working* (Colinsville, MS: Heritage Press Publications, 2014), 54–55.

158 Ibid., 88–89.

159 Colin P. West et al.,"Interventions to Prevent and Reduce Physician Burnout: A Systematic Review and Meta-Analysis," *Lancet* 388, no. 10057 (2016): 2272–2281, accessed September 13, 2017, http://dx.doi.org/10.1016/S0140-6736(16)31279-X.

160 Frankl, Victor, *Man's Search for Meaning* (Boston: Beacon Press, 2014), 105.

individuals will ultimately begin to demonstrate signs and symptoms of burnout, no matter their resilience or capacity to endure stress. Every physician must acknowledge that fact and be prepared to act accordingly. It is crucial to be aware of the tendency to feel there is something inherently wrong with you when experiencing symptoms of burnout. The three dimensions of burnout—emotional exhaustion, depersonalization, and basic job dissatisfaction—can make it very difficult to see meaning in your work.

You may deem staying in your present highly stressful work situation to be a calculated risk you must take. In that event, it is incumbent on you to do everything in your power to labor on the side of this dilemma over which you do exert some level of control. You do have some measure of control over yourself, your resilience, and your resistance to stress. You also always have the ability to remove yourself from the job or establish boundaries with the job/situation.

Here are some recommendations for controlling the paradigm to some degree from the individual standpoint. They include: keeping heart, living in community, loving yourself, connecting with beauty, and developing a spiritual/mindfulness practice.

Beauty will save the world.

—Fyodor Dostoevsky

KEEP HEART

Richard Rohr wrote that 90 percent of people seem to live their lives on cruise control, which equates to being unconscious.[161] That unconsciousness is a lack of awareness of the deepest longings of the heart, reflected by a nearly unspeakable dissatisfaction.

---

161 Richard Rohr, *Falling Upward* (San Francisco: Jossey-Bass, 2011), 90.

Perhaps the most significant difficulty for us physicians is the issue of being so comfortable with putting everything on hold that we live our entire lives on hold. Not being aware of that choice is the worst aspect of the damage we do to ourselves and others. Being on cruise control does not mean that what we do is easy, or that our work does not require a serious depth of thoughtful reasoning. On the contrary, we deal with very difficult complex issues on a daily basis. Our life is on cruise control because we get stuck living in our minds without having heart, without being engaged at the level of the heart and soul. We skim the surface of deep waters not recognizing the turbulence that exists directly below us and within us. Writer and Nobel Prize Laureate William Faulkner said, "The only thing worth writing about is the human heart in conflict with itself." The only way worth living is to engage the heart with all its conflict—whatever that costs. The price for abandoning the heart is too steep.

> *The only way worth living is to engage the heart with all its conflict—whatever that costs. The price for abandoning the heart is too steep.*

John Stone captured this in his poem, "Gaudeamus Igitur":[162]

For the heart will lead
For the head will explain
But the final common pathway is the heart
Whatever kingdom may come
For what matters finally is how the human spirit is spent

---

162 John Stone, "Gaudeamus Igitur," *Journal of the American Medical Association* 249, no. 13 (1983):1741–1742

Everyone has wounds. Often, the deepest of those wounds are inflicted by the people we love and trust the most. In an attempt to avoid ultimate rejection or abandonment, which is perceived emotionally as a type of death, people learn to deny their hearts and wounds for the sake of survival.

The paradox is that people were designed for living a full and abundant life. In fact, John 10:10 tells us, "The thief comes not, but for to steal, and to kill, and to destroy: I am come that they might have life, and that they might have it more abundantly." Yet, too often people stop trusting, stop believing, the desires of their heart. Chip Dodd writes:

> We quit drinking from the waters of emotional and spiritual life. We quit trusting the heart's thirst to be known, seen, fed and expanded. Instead of remaining vulnerable to growth, we resign our hearts to blocking all intrusions of relationship (and, ultimately, love) because of the fear that: (1) relationship is not real, and (2) relationship is real, but will not last.
>
> However they occur, if we do not address these woundings on an emotional and spiritual level by admitting and surrendering to how our hearts are made, they will never heal … We become experts at practicing hopelessness.[163]

The key to thriving, and not just surviving, may be in learning how to burn without burning out:[164] giving, being fully present, suffering disappointment, heartache—even heartbreak—without closing the heart off. You must remain open to what life brings and

---

163 Chip Dodd, *Voice of the Heart: A Call to Full Living*, 2nd ed. (Nashville: Sage Hill Resources, 2014), 16–17.
164 Hence Frankl's quote at the beginning of the chapter.

be willing to feel the hurt, sadness, fear, loneliness, anger, shame, and guilt in order to receive the gifts they bring.

Being unwilling or becoming unwilling to feel these emotions just closes off the joy and everything else that comes from being fully alive. Such unwillingness is an "unforgivable" sin if only because being willing is a prerequisite to healing, as *Christ Healing the Paralytic at the Pool of Bethesda* instructs. Early Christian theologian Irenaeus said the glory of God is man fully alive. So the admonition is to feel your feelings, be willing to tell the truth, and trust the process. Allow God to do the rest, doing for you what you cannot do for yourself. That is what it means to have trust or faith in the process.[165]

Keeping heart requires the willingness to admit powerlessness. It is that simple. Yet it can prove incredibly difficult to live out loud that way. There has to be a willingness to be vulnerable. In a sense, you must be willing to open yourself to the potential of being wounded. But living with openness can awaken you to your humanity, desires, needs, and longings, and allow God the space to move in your life.

> *As it is with medicine, living with openness is a practice. It is not a to-do list that is checked off or a task that is completed. In that sense, there is no method for preventing burnout. Instead, keeping heart is about process, not destination. It is the journey.*

As it is with medicine, living with openness is a practice. It is not a to-do list that is checked off or a task that is completed. In that sense, there *is no method* for preventing burnout. Instead, keeping heart is about process, not

---

165 Ibid., 156.

destination. It is the *journey*. The path is tortuous, more serpentine than direct. It can be difficult work, requiring patience, persistence, and willingness to be engaged. Occasionally, while feeling that no distance is being traversed, the realization comes that tremendous ground has been covered despite being "home."

> We shall not cease from exploration
> And the end of all our exploring
> Will be to arrive where we started
> And know the place for the first time.
>
> —T. S. Eliot[166]

LIVE IN COMMUNITY

If a man has lost a leg or an eye, he knows he has lost a leg or an eye; but if he has lost a self—himself—he cannot know it, because he is no longer there to know it.

—Oliver Sacks, MD

Dike Drummond detailed how to recognize the symptoms of burnout in yourself in his book, *Preventing Physician Burnout: What to Do When Working Harder Isn't Working.*[167] His recommendations for prevention are good ones, and bring a little hope to the possibility that someone can self-diagnose. It is much more likely for people to recognize the symptoms of burnout in themselves if they have suffered through it before.

---

166 Sam Intrator and Megan Scribner, eds., *Leading from Within: Poetry That Sustains the Courage to Lead* (San Francisco; Wiley, 2007), 23.

167 Dike Drummond, *Preventing Physician Burnout: What to Do When Working Harder Isn't Working* (Colinsville, MS: Heritage Press Publications, 2014), 43.

However, one serious difficulty in recommending self-diagnosis lies in the disorienting nature of the dilemma. Physicians must not only recognize the signs or symptoms, but also be honest about their presence and then be willing to ask for help. It is a possible but improbable situation, much like the one faced by Narcissus, the hunter of Greek mythology. Fundamentally he could not recognize himself because he was disoriented.[168] The condition from which he suffered was a result of the curse placed upon him by the Greek goddess Nemesis.[169] By gazing directly into a reflecting pool, staring at his own image, he is, in effect, blinded. He falls in love with his own reflection and suffers from an absurd lack of self-awareness.

As German psychologist Erich Fromm wrote, "The psychological results of alienation are [that] man regresses ... ceases to be productive; that he loses his sense of self, becomes dependent on approval, hence tends to conform and yet to feel insecure; he is dissatisfied, bored, and anxious, and spends most of his energy in the attempt to compensate for or just to cover up this anxiety."[170]

So how difficult is it to recognize the symptoms of burnout in oneself? It is similar to asking those who suffer from schizophrenia to recognize their hallucinations.

A few years ago, a young man was referred to see me after he had been evaluated by an associate. He relayed that he was "pulling material that looks exactly like steel wool" out of his nose almost daily. That activity had been going on for several months. A CT scan ordered by his primary care doctor was normal. His nasal endoscopy was normal. He had no other nasal symptoms. Reviewing his medications, I noted he was on a phenothiazine antipsychotic drug. I

---

168 Craig Malkin, *Rethinking Narcissism: The Secret to Recognizing and Coping with Narcissists* (New York: Harper Collins, 2015), 2–4.

169 Ibid.

170 Eric Fromm, *The Sane Society* (New York: Henry Holt).

asked him if he had ever been diagnosed with schizophrenia, which was not listed in his past medical history (PMH). He replied that he had been previously diagnosed with schizophrenia.

I told him that I would call his psychiatrist because I thought the "symptom" he was experiencing was related to his schizophrenia, and not his nose. Honestly, I was a little afraid he might react harshly, but he merely said, "Oh, okay. I wondered if it might be that. So you think it is a hallucination?"

"Yes, I do," I replied.

His psychiatrist adjusted the medication, and his "steel wool" symptoms resolved. Even though he thought it might be his schizophrenia, he needed help to determine that.

Living in community is vital. By that I mean having a group of friends you trust, and with whom you meet regularly. It is important—and more often than you believe is necessary—to ask these people what they think.

Living in isolation is dangerous. Physicians recognize that principle, but the descent into isolation can occur so insidiously that it can be imperceptible, and the results can be catastrophic. Sam Quinones, in his book about America's opiate epidemic, even identified community as the antidote to heroin addiction.[171]

---

171 Sam Quinones, *Dreamland: The True Tale of America's Opiate Epidemic* (New York: Bloomsbury Press, 2016), 353.

JOHARI'S WINDOW

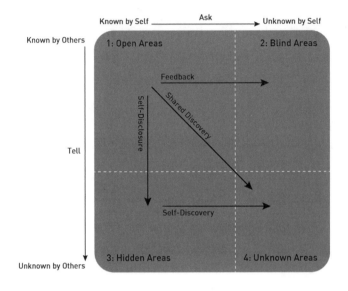

Figure 8-2. Johari's Window

Johari's Window, Figure 8-2,[172] is a heuristic device developed in 1955 by psychologists Joseph Luft and Harrington Ingham. It can inform individuals about how they relate to the world, and how and on what basis other individuals and the world relate to the individual. The model essentially demonstrates the capacity people have to build trust by being honest with one another. It can also help people better understand how well they handle feedback from others. "What is it like to be with me, when there is a rapidly approaching deadline and we have to get the job done?" might be an example of looking for feedback.

Evelyn and I used to play a game called Imaginiff with our children. A representative question from the game might be: Imagine

---

172 The Johari Window, MindTools, accessed May 30, 2017, https://www.mindtools. com/CommSkll/JohariWindow.htm.

if Shawn were an animal, what kind of animal would he be? Then the players would select from four or five options listed on a card. It was more fun with five to ten people, because then everyone would secretly select what kind of animal they believed Shawn was most like, *from their perspective.* Players who matched the majority answer would then move forward on the game board. So, if I saw myself as a tiger, but everyone else viewed me as a weasel, then all those players would move forward, and I would have some self-reflecting to do on how others viewed me. It could be a humbling experience, but it was also a lot of fun.

Everyone occasionally has difficulty determining subjective from objective reality. Everyone needs others to explain how things look from an alternate perspective. Research actually indicates fairly consistently that "most people think of themselves as exceptional and unique. This pervasive phenomenon has been dubbed the 'better than average effect.'"[173] Most of us could use some improvement in our self-awareness. Certainly, it is never perfect. To live in community, where there is the capacity to gather opinions from people who view things from an alternative frame of reference, is the greatest antidote to the malady of disorientation from which we all tend to suffer.

As theologian Thomas Merton explains, "We are not very good at recognizing illusions, least of all the ones we cherish most about ourselves—the ones we are born and raised with and which feed the roots of sin. For most of the people in the world, there is no greater subjective reality than this false self of theirs, which cannot exist. A life devoted to maintaining and expanding this false self, this shadow, is what is called a life of sin."

People need others to be honest with them and to love them enough to confront them and their difficulty, whether that is burnout,

---

173 Craig Malkin, *Rethinking Narcissism* (New York: HarperCollins, 2015), 9.

schizophrenia, narcissism, stress, lack of sleep, lack of motivation, or something else potentially self-destructive and isolating. Burned-out doctors may still ignore the issue and be unwilling to confront their demons, but their chances are improved dramatically by someone willing to move into their life in a loving way.

I am grateful every day that I had and have that in Evelyn. I am also thankful for a group of men—formed after I returned from treatment—who are willing to meet regularly, share the truth about themselves, and listen to me about my often ugly inner world. I am thankful that we hold each other in community, and that we are able to tell each other the truth about our experiences. We all have different problems, but we share having lost heart at some point, and we are willing to talk about it.

What defines a community is completely subjective. For instance, two of the men who worked as counselors at the CPE rode together to work every day in a truck. It took them thirty to forty minutes to make the trip. One of them often said, "Everybody needs a pickup truck." It was Nashville after all, where almost everyone does have a pickup truck. But what he meant was that we all need a place where we can unpack and expose our deepest fears, longings, and desires—our hurts and our anger, our feelings toward another man or woman—and know that nothing will go beyond the cab of that truck. As iron sharpens iron, so one person sharpens another.[174] Therapists refer to this sort of environment as a safe space. I like the idea of the pickup truck.

Self-care is not selfish. You cannot serve from an empty vessel.

—Eleanor Brownn

---

174 Proverbs 27:17, NIV.

LOVE YOURSELF

Compassion has been defined as the emotion experienced when there is concern for the suffering of another coupled with the desire to positively impact that individual's welfare.[175] It seems intuitive that this capacity for compassion would be not only desirable but essential for physicians to have, develop, and continue to cultivate throughout their lifetime of practice.

EMPATHY, SYMPATHY, AND COMPASSION ARE RELATED TO COGNITION AND EMOTION

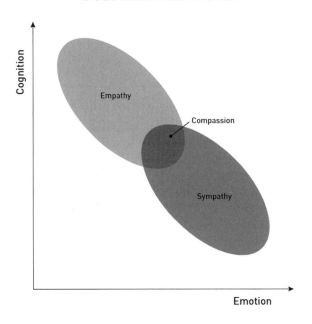

Figure 8-3.

Empathy can be defined as sharing another's emotional state while maintaining awareness that the other person is the source of

---

175 Susanne Leiberg Olga Klimecki and Tania Singer, "Short-Term Compassion Training Increases Prosocial Behavior in a Newly Developed Prosocial Game," *PLoS One* 6, no. 3 (2011): e17798, https://doi.org/10.1371/journal.pone.0017798.

the emotion.[176] Compassion relies on a different neural network than empathy does, but both compassion and empathy appear to be necessary for physician wellness. They are also both associated with high quality patient care (see Figure 8-3).[177]

Conversely, their absence has been shown to increase diagnostic errors.[178] Unfortunately, systematic reviews have reported a significant decline in empathy as medical students progress through medical school, and a high prevalence of burnout among medical undergraduates.[179] Some of this phenomenon may be related to a tendency for empathic resonance associated with the suffering of others in the absence of compassion to activate neural pathways involved in distress. Fortunately, training for compassion has demonstrated a strong positive affect even though it did not lead to the denial of suffering.[180]

Job dissatisfaction relates to a loss of meaning in the work being performed. That feeling of meaninglessness is what Viktor Frankl identified as part of being human, yet he simultaneously recognized that it could be pathogenic and related to feelings of depression, aggression, and addiction. He felt it was secondary to what he referred to as an "existential vacuum."[181] He treated some depressed or suicidal

---

176 P. Kanske et al., "Dissecting the Social Brain: Introducing the EMPAToM to Reveal Distinct Neural Networks and Brain-Behavior Relations for Empathy and Theory of Mind," *NeuroImage* 122 (2015), 6–19.

177 Mohammadreza Hojat, "The Jefferson Scale of Physician Empathy: Development and Preliminary Psychometric Data," *Educational and Psychological Measurement* 61 (April 2001), 349–365.

178 Colin P. West, "Physician Well-Being: Expanding the Triple Aim," *Journal of General Internal Medicine* 31, no. 5 (May 2016), 458—459.

179 Melanie Neumann et al., "Empathy Decline and Its Reasons: A Systematic Review of Studies with Medical Students and Residents," *Academic Medicine* 86, no. 8 (August 2011), 996–1009.

180 Olga M. Klimecki et al., "Functional Neural Plasticity and Associated Changes in Positive Affect after Compassion Training," *Cerebral Cortex* 23, no. 7 (July 2013), 1552–1561, doi:10.1093/cercor/bhs142.

181 Viktor Frankl, *Man's Search for Meaning* (Boston: Beacon Press), 133–137.

patients by having them volunteer. The interjection of meaning and purpose into their lives from volunteering was restorative.

Practically, then, how does one cognitively set out to find meaning? If volunteering helped interject meaning and purpose back into the lives of Dr. Frankl's depressed patients, it would seem to follow that physicians would be very resistant to a loss of meaning in work. Practicing medicine is so steeped in deep fundamental meaning, it is problematic to figure out how one would set out to lose meaning while laboring as a doctor. Has an existential vacuum been unwittingly created?

The issues of job-related burnout do not occur in a milieu devoid of individual variability and susceptibility. While the data on the numbers of physicians experiencing burnout point to organizational culpability as the prime mover, individual variables such as personality, level of education, marital status, the need for approval, need for control, capacity for emotional regulation, history of trauma, family of origin issues, and the degree of spiritual development have an impact on the amount of individual resilience. These are some of the factors that can make a physician more or less susceptible to burnout.[182]

In truth, I still carry a sense of shame about not being tough enough to take whatever was dished out in the course of practicing my profession and surviving my childhood. That is one aspect of my experience I felt most acutely. I still run the scenarios in my mind of how I could have done X, Y, or Z differently. I often find myself thinking, "I should have . . . " At the end of that road is the blame I place on myself.

---

182 Christina Maslach, *Burnout: The Cost of Caring* (Los Altos, CA: Malor Books, 2003), 93–120.

All of this thinking is reinforced by my training. That is part of the reason I ended up where I did: in therapy for PTSD-related depression resulting not just from one particular episode, but a lifetime accumulation of emotional detritus I had not dealt with adequately, if at all. While there is an argument to be made that I succumbed to burnout because of some inherent defect or weakness, the staggering figures related to burnout suggest that there are structural, organizational, even systemic problems in the process of training and practice that deserve investigation and redress. A fundamental attribution error refers to the tendency to overestimate personal factors and underestimate external or situational ones when explaining behavior.[183] Identifying and enhancing the tools available for individual physicians to increase resilience and decrease stress to mitigate burnout is necessary but *not* sufficient. Institutional and organizational change is an imperative.

Mined from the well of my own experience, compassion for ourselves can be the place where we feel it is most difficult to practice empathy or compassion. Grace is by definition unmerited favor. Grace is what a merciful, loving God bestows. How is it even fathomable, then, for us to extend grace to ourselves? How do we even grant ourselves mercy and favor knowing that we do not deserve these gifts? The whole miserable mess of life is our own fault, our responsibility: the ingratitude, the selfishness, the inappropriate remarks, the deceit, the lack of mercy, the judgment of others.

The second part of the second greatest commandment in Luke 10:27, to love ... "as yourself,"[184] can be agonizingly difficult to apply. I often entertain the idea that doing so is an attempt to escape

---

183 Ibid.,16.

184 Jesus referred to these laws as the "greatest/foremost and the second being like the first" in Mark 12:29–31.

responsibility for my actions. That notion is often seconded by a cadre of people who seem unwilling to allow me the grace and mercy sufficient to forgive myself. My inner voice argues that by forgiving myself I am not taking responsibility.[185] It is a wicked path to navigate: a complete lack of self-compassion versus an over-indulgent narcissistic tendency to have it be all about me.

There is a middle path.

The principal issue is not with the people in your life. Whether they be friends, relatives, enemies, church leaders, or bystanders—you do not need permission from anyone to practice compassion for, or exhibit empathy toward, anyone else. However, if you are like me, you only have the capacity to practice compassion to the extent you are able to extend it toward yourself. Hence, there is an argument that you do not need anyone's permission for the compassion you extend toward yourself either.

Included in the concept of loving yourself is caring for your own physical needs. The need for you, as a human being, to recognize your requirement for sufficient sleep, regular exercise, and proper nutrition is obvious. There is a tendency to sacrifice such needs when stress and time constraints begin to dictate the tempo of life. We have a responsibility to care for ourselves.[186]

The next two concepts of connecting with beauty and developing a spiritual/mindfulness practice greatly assist in the practice of self-compassion, or loving oneself.

---

185 See Inner Voice discussion on page 28.

186 Tait D. Shanafelt, Lotte N. Dyrbye, and Colin P. West, "Addressing Physician Burnout: The Way Forward," *Journal of the American Medical Association* 317, no. 9 (2017): 901–902.

CONNECT WITH BEAUTY

Beauty is to the spirit what food is to the flesh. A glimpse of it in a young face, say, or an echo of it in a song fills an emptiness in you that nothing else under the sun can.

—Frederick Buechner

There is a plethora of data supporting improvement in psychological functioning with various forms of creative work, art, and/or art therapy.[187] Creativity has been demonstrated to be a means of cultivating positive psychological functioning.[188] Physicians have taken notice, and are beginning to engage their creative side, recognizing its healing power.[189] Some medical schools and residency training programs have incorporated communal art viewing as well as art classes as a way to increase sensitivity, discuss end-of-life issues, encourage team building, and facilitate collaboration. "Incorporating the humanities into medical education has been shown to increase empathy, awareness, and sensitivity to the art of medicine."[190]

Listening to Mozart, painting a landscape, throwing pottery, dancing, making a dulcimer, writing or reading poetry, skiing in the Rockies, writing narrative or prose, hiking Elephant Back Loop trail

---

187 Caroline Alexander, "Behind the Mask: Revealing the Trauma of War," *National Geographic*, May 19, 2015.

188 Tamlin S. Conner, Colin G. DeYoung, and Paul J. Silvia, "Everyday Creative Activity as a Path to Flourishing," *The Journal of Positive Psychology*, pub. online November 17, 2016, doi:10.1080/17439760.2016.1257049.

189 Anokhi Saklecha, "Creativity in Medicine: A Burned Out ER Physician Turns to Art," *Op-(m)ed* (blog) at Doximity, https://opmed.doximity.com/about-9b9265b6b950.

190 Jo Marie Riley, Jeffrey Ring, and Linda Duke, "Visual Thinking Strategies: A New Role for Art in Medical Education," *Family Medicine* 37, no. 4 (April 2005): 250–252; Casey Lesser, "Why Med Schools Are Requiring Art Classes," ART SY, Aug 21, 2017, accessed September 3, 2017, https://www.artsy.net/article/artsy-editorial-med-schools-requiring-art-classes/amp.

in Yellowstone, and a host of similar activities, all have the capacity to transport and draw from people emotions they might have buried. These endeavors are shrouded with elements of beauty, or the act of creating. Sometimes, they encompass both beauty and creation. Therein lies their potential to reinvigorate. A creative act can call forth a sense of order and truth, reflections of beauty out of chaos. It is redemptive.[191] We are buying back a little piece of the world and a little of ourselves at the same time.

Steven Curtis Chapman has five Grammy Awards and a plethora of Gospel Music Association Dove Awards, and has sold more than ten million albums. His family suffered the tragic death of his youngest daughter, Maria Sue, in May 2008. Steven recently wrote, "I began to turn to my faithful friend, music, to process what I was thinking and feeling. Music became a way to voice my laments, questions, fears, and hopes."[192]

One of my favorite evangelists was fond of saying he did not wish to "whittle on God's end of the stick." Redemptive, creative acts are our end of the stick. Psalm 19 spurs people to see Him in what He created. Humankind was given dominion over His creation. It is our part of God's work in which we attempt to envision, and then create, a world from what He has given us.

When I began to study classical paintings, following my recovery, I was aware enough to ask the questions, What am I feeling? What is the sadness about? What is the hurt about? … the loneliness? … the guilt and the gladness? The experience always brought me to some part of my story and informed me about me. Merton said it this way, "Art enables us to find ourselves and lose ourselves at the same time."

191 Leland Ryken, ed., *The Christian Imagination: The Practice of Faith in Literature and Writing* (New York: Shaw Books/Penguin Random House, 2002), 84–89.

192 Steven Curtis Chapman, *Between Heaven and the Real World: My Story,* with Ken Abraham (Grand Rapids: Revell Books, 2017), 369.

Connecting with beauty through art has enabled me to see beauty in other places I was overlooking, or had just grown too cynical, jaded, or perhaps, too ill to see. The ability to discern can inform every area of your life if you allow it. When you are present enough to look observantly, you can find order, truth, beauty, and, as a consequence, compassion in the ugliest of circumstances. Theologian William Dyrness wrote, "Here is where the biblical view and the Greek view stand in the greatest possible contrast. In the Old Testament, an object or event is not beautiful because it conforms to a formal ideal but because it reflects in its small way the wholeness of the created order."[193] The masters of the late Renaissance period, particularly Rembrandt, typified this idea of beauty being reflected in realism.

The limbic system response to all we see and experience as physicians has consequences that can adversely affect us, a factor I discussed in some detail in chapter 1, "My Fall and Redemption." The humanities have a way of making us feel more human.

DEVELOP A SPIRITUAL/MINDFULNESS PRACTICE

If, as Maslach elucidated, burnout is truly an "erosion of the human soul,"[194] and the soul is the truth of who I am,[195] then burnout can be thought of as an *erosion of who I am*. The symptoms of emotional exhaustion, depersonalization, and

> *Burnout reveals a soul in search of itself.*

---

193 William Dyrness, *Visual Faith: Art, Theology and Worship in Dialogue* (Grand Rapids: Baker Book House, 2001), 81.

194 Christina Maslach and Michael P. Leiter, *The Truth about Burnout: How Organizations Cause Personal Stress and What to Do about It* (San Francisco: Jossey-Bass, Inc., 1997), 17.

195 A concept of spiritual teacher, author, and lecturer Marianne Williamson.

loss of a sense of accomplishment can be treated, but, at its root, *burnout reveals a soul in search of itself.*

It is axiomatic that in order to give something a person must first possess it. To give of myself, in other words, I must first be in possession of my *self*, which is another way of saying that I must know, deep down, who I am. If burnout is an erosion of the soul, then nurturing the soul, replenishing, and feeding it has to be a critical aspect of prevention and recovery. Directing a person's soul to activities, experiences, and people that encourage the development or re-establishment of a sense of values, dignity, and will are effective ways to ameliorate this dilemma in the individual. This is the essence of spirituality.

Spirituality concerns the soul or spirit. Religion has more to do with a particular system of belief or worship. As a result, religion tends to involve itself with the discussion of rules. Are rules important? Yes, but faith, hope, and love are more important.[196] Jesus railed against the religious elite for tithing spices while leaving out the "weightier matters," which were also law. He identified these weightier matters as justice, mercy, and faith.[197]

I disobeyed my parents and often suffered for it, not only because I was sometimes punished, but also because the rule was there to protect me and, in disobeying it, I ended up experiencing the difficulty from which they tried to protect me. However, I don't ever recall being enamored by their rules and guidelines. It was their love, their patience, their faithfulness and generosity toward me that helped to transform me. Richard Rohr wrote: "The people who know

196 I Cor 13:13.
197 Matthew 23:23.

God well—mystics, hermits, prayerful people, those who risk every-thing to find God—always meet a lover, not a dictator."[198]

It is also evident, then, that the specific aspects and nature of the spiritual search for the self will be individualized. The journey can be encouraged. The embarkation point can be alluded to, but the specific path is peculiar.

MINDFULNESS

> *All of humanity's problems stem from man's*
> *inability to sit quietly in a room alone.*
>
> ### —Blaise Pascal

Busyness is often a subconsciously purposeful distraction from being truly present. We don't have any desire to be alone with ourselves in a room. There are techniques or practices—which are effective strategies for allowing one to develop presence in a way that has been demonstrated to promote healing—that reduce stress and anxiety and promote a sense of acceptance.[199]

Contemplative prayer and centering prayer can be viewed within the wider tradition of Christian meditative practices. Con-templative prayer is described as nondual consciousness, or a way of being in presence, or objectless awareness, and is closely connected to centering prayer. There is both an eastern and a western mystical

---

198 Richard Rohr, *Everything Belongs: The Gift of Contemplative Prayer* (New York: The Crossroad Publishing Co., 2013).

199 Bassam Khoury et al., "Mindfulness-Based Stress Reduction for Healthy Individu-als: A Meta-Analysis," *Journal of Psychosomatic Research* 78, no. 6 (June 2015): 519–528.

tradition of contemplative prayer that dates back to the Desert Fathers in the third century.[200]

Mindfulness is "awareness of present experience with acceptance."[201] It has also been described as nonjudgmental attention to experiences in the present moment.[202] Mindfulness is a focus of *attention* on something like the breath or a mantra. Centering prayer has at its core a focus of *intention* toward God, described as heartfulness. These practices begin to sound a lot alike, though contemplative prayer and centering prayer have not been scientifically studied to the same extent as mindfulness.

Mindfulness-based stress reduction (MBSR) techniques have demonstrated the ability to reduce symptoms of burnout in health care professionals.[203] MBSR was developed by Jon Kabat-Zinn, who placed the Buddhist teachings on meditation and mindfulness into a scientific context, removing the elements of religion. While there is a lot of evidence that this type of mindfulness training effects significant positive changes when performed over a long period of time, there is also evidence that positive changes occur relatively quickly with this type of contemplative training.[204]

---

200 See bibliography: Bourgeault, Foster, Merton, and Rohr.

201 Paul Gilbert, *The Compassionate Mind: A New Approach to Life's Challenges* (Oakland: New Harbinger Press, 2009).

202 Jon Kabat-Zinn, "An Outpatient Program in Behavioral Medicine for Chronic Pain Patients Based on the Practice of Mindfulness Meditation: Theoretical Considerations and Preliminary Results," *General Hospital Psychiatry* 4, no. 1 (April 1982): 33–47.

203 A. Amutio et al., "Acceptability and Effectiveness of a Long-Term Educational Intervention to Reduce Physicians' Stress Related Conditions," *Journal of Continuing Education in Health Professionals* 35, no. 4 (2015), 255–260.

204 Boris Bornemann et al., "Differential Changes in Self-Reported Aspects of Interoceptive Awareness through 3 Months of Contemplative Training," *Frontiers in Psychology* 5, article 1504 (pub. online January 6, 2015), 1–13; Susanne Leiberg, Olga Klimecki, and Tania Singer, "Short-Term Compassion Training Increases Prosocial Behavior in a Newly Developed Prosocial Game," *PLoS One* 6, no. 3: e 17798, https://doi.org/10.1371/journal.pone.0017798.

Conceptually, these practices are radical departures from what had been my normal way of functioning, but I am learning to live and to be different. After all, it is practice, not perfection, that is important.

One of the primary benefits of these meditative practices, for me, has been a growing awareness of when I need to "let go." I find it much easier to assume a non-egoic or self-emptying posture when I am able to practice presence or awareness using these methods.[205]

Barry Kerzin, an American-trained physician and Buddhist monk, is the personal physician to the Dalai Lama. Following the tragic death of his wife in 1983, Kerzin worked as an assistant professor of medicine at the University of Washington School of Medicine for approximately four years. In 1988, he took what was to be a six-month leave of absence to go to Dharamsala, India, but he has essentially remained there ever since. I had the opportunity to meet him and hear him speak at the White Coat Ceremony for incoming medical students at the University of Louisville in the late summer of 2016. My son is in the class of 2020.

I happened to be staying at the same hotel as Dr. Kerzin, and recognized him as he entered the lobby. We spoke for just a few minutes, and what captured me immediately about him was a gentle equanimity of spirit. Despite the fact that I had interrupted him, he gave me his full attention and listened with genuine curiosity to my prattle about how interested I was in his work.

Dr. Kerzin has spoken often and at length about the need for more compassion in the practice of medicine. "Approaching the cultivation of compassion from many paths ensures a better result. Not only can we directly practice compassion, we can also indirectly practice compassion. This dual approach maximizes the cultivation

---

205 Philippians 2:7.

of compassion," he wrote in 2013.[206] He also writes of generosity, honesty, forgiveness, patience, perseverance, and concentration, and how these can be practiced with a focused, non-distracted mind. These characteristics or qualities can be a means of indirectly practicing compassion. Mindfulness is not only a way of developing compassion, but also a method of enhancing these other indirect means of cultivating compassion.

There is little doubt that compassion training, a contemplative mindset, centering prayer, and/or mindfulness-based stress reduction has a role in the development of a more appropriate empathic response to suffering and reducing stress-related responses to that suffering. Yet, at least with respect to medical students and residents, "Limited data are available regarding how to best address trainee burnout, but multi-pronged efforts, with attention to culture, the learning and work environment and individual behaviors [sic] are needed to promote trainees' wellness and to help those in distress."[207] There is less data on those in practice, but certainly it could be argued that the approach to burnout must be multifaceted even though the facets may look a little different once the physician is out of medical school or residency.

Keeping heart, living in community, loving yourself, connecting with beauty, and having a spiritual and mindfulness practice—each works independently, and together they promote wellness. Mindfulness will assist in compassion toward oneself and the development of awareness, for example. A spiritual practice can help one to develop

---

206 Barry Kerzin, "Cultivating Alternative Paths to Compassion: Generosity, Forgiveness, and Patience," in *Compassion. Bridging Practice and Science*, edited by Tania Singer and Matthias Bolz (Munich, Germany: Max Planck Society, 2013), e-book available at www.compassion-training.org/?lang.

207 Liselotte Dyrbye and Tait Shanafelt, "A Narrative Review on Burnout Experienced by Medical Students and Residents," *Medical Education* 50, no. 1 (January 2016), 132–149.

purpose and meaning within a broader context than that of the self. Having a group of friends with whom I can truly be honest and open, trusting them with the truth of who I am and what I am feeling, helps me keep heart as a result of living in community. They give me an important perspective on the experience of being with me. Connecting with beauty allows me to access my feelings in a way I may not have been able to before and gives me opportunities to practice sharing those feelings with others. The essence of all of these practices is nourishment of the soul, which is in search of itself.

But what of those other facets that need to be addressed? What of the organizational response to suffering and physician burnout? Let's look at that aspect of well-being next.

FIND YOUR
HEART

You are no longer to supply the people with straw for making bricks; let them go and gather their own straw. But require them to make the same number of bricks as before; don't reduce the quota. They are lazy; that is why they are crying out, "Let us go and sacrifice to our God."[208]

—Exodus 5:7–8

---

208 Exodus 5:7–8 (NIV).

THE ORGANIZATIONAL RESPONSE

Pharaoh's demand that the Israelites make the same number of bricks while dramatically increasing their difficulty in doing so may be the first example of poor leadership giving rise to increased organizational stress. I recently attended a Harvard course on compassion in practice codirected by Dr. Beth Lown. It was about focused attempts to achieve better outcomes by increasing resilience and improving collaboration. Over 250 health care professionals attended. The great preponderance of attendees were physicians. I was the only surgeon.

Dr. Lown, an associate professor of medicine at Harvard, is also the medical director of the Schwartz Center for Compassionate Healthcare in Boston. During the conference, Lown discussed the fact that compassion is a universal human response to suffering that organizations can extinguish.[209] While medical schools and residency programs are undoubtedly aware of the burnout dilemma and its associated effects on quality, the organizational response has been lethargic at best, but certainly culpable at least.

The prevalence of burnout in physicians speaks much more about the current state of health care and the conditions under which doctors practice than it does about the physicians themselves.[210] The data is relatively consistent in viewing burnout as an organizational issue that needs to be addressed on that level.[211] Research has indicated dissatisfaction and burnout may be ameliorated by addressing issues related to workflow, communication, and taking clinicians' quality

---

209 Beth Lown, "Activating Compassion: Implementing a Framework for Compassionate, Collaborative Healthcare," (plenary presentation at Harvard Medical School "Compassion in Practice" course, Boston, Massachusetts, October 28, 2016).

210 Christina Maslach and Michael P. Leiter, *The Truth about Burnout: How Organizations Cause Personal Stress and What to Do about It* (San Francisco: Jossey-Bass, 1997), 21.

211 Ibid., 18.

concerns seriously.[212] Institutional support of facilitated small groups incorporating multiple elements such as mindfulness, reflection, and sharing decreased overall rates of burnout.[213] It should be noted that this support included paying for the physicians' time to participate, which not only encourages participation but reflects the organization's commitment to, and support of, the medical staff.

Comprehensive recommendations for institutions should at least include the following steps, as modified from Mark Linzer et al.:[214]

1. Institutional metrics on physician well-being and burnout need to be routine. We know that what is measured generally improves. The structural and relational environment of every organization is somewhat unique. Routine monitoring of the level of emotional exhaustion, depersonalization, and loss of meaning in the work of physicians would allow identification of strategies to address the dimension(s) of the burnout syndrome, which appeared to be deteriorating. Additionally, there would be objective evidence of either improvement or further deterioration once strategies were implemented to combat the decline in the dimension(s) previously identified.

2. Physician self-care needs to be considered an important aspect of medical professionalism. Rishi Sikka, Julianne

---

212 Mark Linzer et al., "A Cluster Randomized Trial of Interventions to Improve Work Conditions and Clinician Burnout in Primary Care: Results from the Healthy Work Place (HWP) Study," *Journal of General Internal Medicine* 30, no. 8 (August 2015), 1105–1111.

213 Colin P. West et al., "Intervention to Promote Physician Well-Being, Job Satisfaction, and Professionalism: A Randomized Clinical Trial," *JAMA Internal Medicine* 174, no. 4 (April 2014), 527–533.

214 Mark Linzer et al., "10 Bold Steps to Prevent Burnout in General Internal Medicine," *Journal of General Internal Medicine* 29, no. 1 (January 2014): 18–20.

Morath, and Lucian Leape advocate for a modification of the *triple aim* of health care as detailed by Donald Berwick,[215] which they referred to as the *quadruple aim*.[216] This expands the concept that improving the experience of care, the health of populations, and lowering the cost of health care, are fundamentally related to the meaning that physicians find in performing their work. Programs and initiatives that aid physicians in discovering or retaining joy and meaning in their work could be justifiably incorporated as part of a quality improvement program. Mindfulness-based stress reduction techniques need to be taught and incorporated into medical training and medical staff activities. Students and residents should be encouraged to engage professional coaches or counselors as part of their training.[217]

3.   Electronic health record (EHR) stress relief that incorporates a variety of strategies unique to individual practices and physicians is one of the primary ways organizational clout can be effectively utilized to mitigate burnout. Few physicians go into medicine to be data entry clerks. Customized templates with individual programmability, communication with physicians on the particular needs of different specialties, scribes, and taking complaints regarding intrusion and workflow seriously can be of great value in

215 Donald M. Berwick, Thomas W. Nolan, and John Whittington, "The Triple Aim: Care, Health and Cost," *Health Affairs* 27, no. 3 (May 2008), 759–769.

216 Rishi Sikka, Julianne M. Morath, and Lucian Leape, "The Quadruple Aim: Care, Health, Cost and Meaning in Work," (editorial), *BMJ Quality and Safety* 24, no. 10 (October 2015), 608–610.

217 Gail Gazelle, Jane M. Liebschutz, and Helen Riess, "Physician Burnout: Coaching a Way Out," *Journal of General Internal Medicine* 30, no. 4 (April 2015): 508–513.

reducing organizational stress. Dike Drummond places the mitigation of EHR-related strain under personal stress relief tools, and he has really good suggestions for how to address it on an individual basis.[218] EHR issues really cross the spectrum as both organizational stress and individual stress. As a result, these EHR issues need to be addressed both individually and institutionally.

To seriously address the issue definitively, we need a bold new initiative or paradigm shift on how physicians are paid. *Meaningful use* needs to function in a manner reflective of its name. I routinely produce a twelve-page note when a paragraph would be better, all because it is required for payment. It is preposterous, burdensome, and time consuming. The production of this type of note only impairs communication. It does not facilitate it. Bullet counting needs to disappear. The computer/EHR is not the problem as much as the way in which we have been enslaved to utilize it.

> *The production of this type of note only impairs communication. It does not facilitate it. Bullet counting needs to disappear. The computer/EHR is not the problem as much as the way in which we have been enslaved to utilize it.*

Is it the musings of a lunatic to wonder what would result if we were to design the progress and/or office visit note around the information physicians think is pertinent? We do not do our profession or our patients any service by being complicit in this charade.

---

218 Dike Drummond, *Stop Physician Burnout: What to Do When Working Harder Isn't Working* (Colinsville, MS: Heritage Press Publications, 2014), 91–99.

These types of solutions are more long-term in nature, however. In the interim, limiting administrative stress will depend more on the hospital system or institution where one works, and the application of the individual tools Drummond recommends. A realistic assessment indicates that these are the areas over which we exert more influence and thus will meet with more immediate returns.

4. Staffing ratios, visit duration, and reasonable panel sizes must be maintained. Work conditions must be improved in clinics and offices, especially those that deal with minority or disenfranchised populations. These clinics tend to be shackled with too much to do and too little with which to accomplish it. Clinics and offices need to incorporate some measure of flexibility to enable physicians to control and customize their schedules. To accomplish this, opportunities for part-time positions and job sharing should be provided. The goal is to address the environmental factors that can lead to burnout over time. One health system recently implemented shadowing as a part of its physician wellness program. Consultants shadowed more than fifteen physicians. One key finding led to changes that helped offload non-physician work to other staff. [219]

5. Compassion and collaboration must be valued at all organizational levels. Values-based employment models that take into account these types of skills are important to consider. Measurement of compassion throughout the

---

219 Sara Berg, "Shadowing Reveals More Efficient Way to Practice Medicine," AMA Wire, Aug 28, 2017, accessed September 3, 2017, https://wire.ama-assn.org/life-career/shadowing-reveals-more-efficient-ways-practice-medicine?utm.

continuum of care will allow the valuation and reward of compassionate care.[220]

All of these recommendations need to be incorporated where appropriate to the training of physicians. The value we say we place on compassion and empathy needs to be intentionally reflected in how students and residents are mentored and taught. Courses that foster the development of competence in narrative medicine need to be employed.

Organizations may help ameliorate the stress in today's medical work environment. Indeed, they have an ethical imperative to do so. It is evident, however, from the statistics regarding physician burnout, that they are more efficient at extinguishing compassion than developing it. It is left to individual souls who possess compassion to help develop it in others and move within their organizations to institute changes and begin to create a culture that values and fosters compassion.

Medical institutions are in dire need of physicians who are willing to take a stand and demand that the medical work environment improves for the good of the patient, the caregiver, and the health care system. It is imperative that physician well-being becomes a principal concern. It is a public health crisis that needs to be addressed now.

---

220 B. A. Lown, S. J. Muncer, and R. Chadwick, "Can Compassionate Healthcare Be Measured? The Schwartz Center Compassionate Care Scale," *Patient Education and Counseling* 98, no. 8 (August 2015), 1005–1010.

CONCLUSION

Nothing can save you, but writing.

—Charles Bukowski

Studies indicate that over 50 percent of physicians in the United States are suffering from at least one symptom of burnout.[221] If you are a doctor, there is more than an even chance you exhibit some degree of burnout. There are a myriad ways burnout can manifest itself if left unabated: alcoholism, addiction, suicide, disruptive behavior, affairs, acting out, raging, depression, obsessive-compulsive behaviors, and so on. This is a crisis on a personal, professional, public health, and health system level.

It needs to be noted, however, that burnout is not limited to medical professionals. The same dilemma occurs in the corporate world. Herbert Freudenberger first documented burnout. He described it in the staff of newly innovated free clinics originally conceived in Haight-Ashbury in the 1960s.[222] Christina Maslach and Michael Leiter, in the late 1990s, documented that burnout had become "more widespread," and a major issue in occupations

---

221 Tait D. Shanafelt et al., "Changes in Burnout and Satisfaction with Work-Life Balance in Physicians and the General US Working Population between 2011 and 2014," *Mayo Clinic Proceedings* 90, no. 12 (December 2015): 1600–1613, accessed June 15, 2017, http://www.mayoclinicproceedings.org/article/S0025-6196(15)00716-8/abstract.

222 Herbert Freudenberger, "Staff Burn-Out," *Journal of Social Issues* 30, no. 1 (January 1974).

other than those just focused on human services.[223] While the rates of burnout among physicians and medical trainees have increased dramatically, burnout rates for other executives and professionals have not necessarily diminished.

On the positive side, it might be relatively easy to find colleagues who can identify with your feelings no matter where you work. Find them! Develop a cadre of friends with whom you can be real. If you are exhibiting signs or symptoms of burnout, it is imperative you immediately begin to decrease your stress and increase your resilience. I would strongly urge you to seek professional help.

> *If you are exhibiting signs or symptoms of burnout, it is imperative you immediately begin to decrease your stress and increase your resilience. I would strongly urge you to seek professional help.*

If you have not been affected yet—awesome. Start a preventative maintenance program. Even if you are not having signs or symptoms of burnout, increasing your resilience and making attempts to mitigate developing burnout makes a lot of sense, given the hazards of our profession. If you are a physician leader, start a discussion group on this issue at whatever level you serve. That will help to build a sense of community.

Take some time to remember what led you to choose medicine as a career and develop a way to tap into that meaning. It seems easy for that to get lost in day-to-day minutiae. Perhaps it is time for a career change. Maybe it is not, but you have to be willing to

---

223 Christina Maslach and Michael P. Leiter, *The Truth about Burnout: How Organizations Cause Personal Stress and What to Do about It* (San Francisco: Jossey-Bass, 1997).

ask the difficult questions and to make decisions based on how you honestly answer those questions. I would caution against making a quick judgment, however. Steps toward a career change in general are more favorably executed if well planned, thoughtful, and deliberate.

Look for the activities outside of medicine that bring you the greatest joy. Do them regularly. Schedule them; do not just fit them in. Make work fit in around them. This can take great effort. Evelyn and I go out to dinner regularly. We are in church three times a week. We average a twelve- to fifteen-mile bike ride on a local trail once or twice a week. There are a group of men, who are all physicians in recovery, with whom I meet just to talk about life. We try to meet once a week, and often we do. Sometimes we go several weeks without meeting because life happens. I lift with a personal trainer twice a week. I arrange my operating room schedule and office around those two hours. I consider them sacrosanct. Meditating and practicing centering prayer is critical for me to maintain a sense of presence. I struggle to find time, but endeavor to practice at least ten to fifteen minutes a day. When I am able to do some sort of MBSR, which, for me, is centering prayer, it is always a better day. I strive to go on a mission trip[224] to a third world country once a year, in part because those experiences remind me of why I became a physician, and help me to find meaning in my work.

Finding beauty in everyday life can help to cultivate a healthy emotional life. I found my heart's voice in art from the Renaissance. The word *Renaissance* is derived from a French word, which means "rebirth." You may discover your heart in origami, hiking, playing guitar, painting, travel, sculpting, meditating, reading scripture,

---

224 I personally prefer to participate in organizations that have a commitment to a local area or region, that exhibit sustained effort there, and that intimately involves the community and its leaders.

mountain climbing, or a combination of these, but the heart must be found or born again. The soul in search of itself must have the head firmly rooted in the heart. Chronicling that search can be a helpful adjunct.

Writing for me has been restorative, therapeutic, illuminating, informative—and painful. Yet those words seem like trifles in describing what the process of writing has meant to me in my soul. There is an inner life we all possess. Reflection and creativity imbued with a sense of mystery flow out and onto the page in writing. In that process the writer and the reader discover things together. It is intimate. In the process of finding our way through that dark night of the soul, to which St. John of the Cross refers in his medieval classic, we discover meaning. Writing is revelatory as much to ourselves as it is to others.

Writer Pat Schneider discusses that private inner life in her book *How the Light Gets In: Writing as a Spiritual Practice*: "In writing we see, sometimes with fear and trembling, who we have been, who we really are, and we glimpse now and then who we might become."[225] I think it's no accident that the apostle Paul implored us to work out our own salvation with fear and trembling.[226] Perhaps that is one reason he wrote; he was working out his salvation.

All that you can give back to God, or, in fact, offer to anyone else, is your true self—who you really are. That search for healing or wholeness is not ancillary; it is central. In fact, I am not done. I am still becoming, struggling, searching. That is my journey.

---

225 Pat Schneider, *How the Light Gets In: Writing as a Spiritual Practice* (NY: Oxford University Press, 2013), 99.

226 Philippians 2:12.

FIND YOUR
HEART

- ☐ Outline a plan to implement the individual recommendations for burnout.

- ☐ What is your plan for attempting to address some of the organizational recommendations to mitigate burnout?

- ☐ Mindfulness-based stress reduction, centering prayer, and other types of meditative practices trace their origins to spiritual traditions. This may be a comfortable or an uncomfortable truth. Have curiosity about that. Is the comfort/discomfort you perceive fear, sadness, anger, hurt, gladness, guilt, or shame? What is that about? Would it increase or decrease the likelihood that you would employ one of practices?

- ☐ Maslach said burnout was an erosion of the soul. It what sense do you feel that erosion? Considering the recommendations for mitigating burnout, which one do you feel is most important for you in stopping the erosion of who you are?

- ☐ How do you plan on incorporating beauty and/or creativity into your life?

BIBLIOGRAPHY

Bourgeault, Cynthia. *Centering Prayer and Inner Awakening* (Lanham, MD: Cowley Publications, 2004); *The Heart of Centering Prayer: Nondual Christianity in Theory and Practice*. Boulder, CO: Shambhala Publications, 2016.

Bromiley, G. W. ed. *International Standard Bible Encyclopedia*, vols. 1–4. Grand Rapids, Michigan: Eerdmans, 1979.

Brown, Brené. *I Thought It Was Just Me (But It Isn't): Making the Journey from "What Will People Think?" to "I Am Enough."* New York: Avery (Penguin Random House), 2007.

Caldwell, C. G. *Truth Commentary: Luke*. Bowling Green, Kentucky: Guardian of Truth Foundation, 2011.

Chapman, Steven Curtis. *Between Heaven and the Real World: My Story*. With Ken Abraham. Grand Rapids, Michigan: Revell Books, 2017.

Charon, Rita, Sayantani DasGupta, Nellie Hermann, Craig Irvine, Eric R. Marcus, Edgar Rivera Colón, Danielle Spencer, and Maura Spiegel. *The Principles and Practice of Narrative Medicine*. New York: Oxford University Press, 2017.

Courtois Christine and Julian Ford, editors, *Treating Complex Traumatic Stress Disorders: Scientific Foundations and Therapeutic Models* (New York: Guilford 2009).

Cozolino, Louis. *The Neuroscience of Psychotherapy: Healing the Social Brain*. New York: W. W. Norton, 2010.

Dodd, Chip. *The Voice of the Heart: A Call to Full Living*. 2nd ed. Nashville, Tennessee: Sage Hill Resources, 2014.

Drummond, Dike. *Stop Physician Burnout: What to Do When Working Harder Isn't Working*. Colinsville, Mississippi: Heritage Press Publications, 2014.

Dyrness, William. *Visual Faith: Art, Theology and Worship in Dialogue*. Grand Rapids, Michigan: Baker Academic, 2001.

Eldredge, John. *Fathered by God: Learning What Your Dad Could Never Teach You*. Nashville, Tennessee: Thomas Nelson, 2009; *Waking the Dead: The Glory of a Heart Fully Alive*. Nashville, Tennessee: Thomas Nelson, 2003; *Wild at Heart: Discovering the Secret of a Man's Soul*. Nashville, Tennessee: Thomas Nelson, 2001.

Foster, Richard. *Celebration of Discipline: The Path to Spiritual Growth*. New York: HarperCollins, 1978.

Frankl, Victor. *Man's Search for Meaning*. Boston, Massachusetts: Beacon Press, 2014.

Intrator, Sam and Megan Scribner, eds. *Leading from Within: Poetry That Sustains the Courage to Lead*. San Francisco, California: Jossey-Bass (Wiley), 2007.

Kalanithi, Paul. *When Breath Becomes Air*. New York: Random House, 2016.

Keating, Thomas, *Open Mind, Open Heart* (London: Bloomsbury, 2006).

Keil, C. F. and Delitzsch, F. *Commentary on the Old Testament*, vols. 1–4. Grand Rapids, Michigan: Eerdmans, 1971.

King, Daniel. *Truth Commentary: John*. Bowling Green, Kentucky: Guardian of Truth Foundation, 1998.

L'Engle, Madeleine. *Walking on Water: Reflections on Faith and Art*. Wheaton, Illinois: Harold Shaw, 1980.

Malkin, Craig. *Rethinking Narcissism: The Secret to Recognizing and Coping with Narcissists.* New York: HarperCollins, 2015.

Manning, Brennan. *The Ragamuffin Gospel.* New York: Multnomah Books, 2005.

Maslach, Christina. *Burnout: The Cost of Caring.* Los Altos, California: Malor Books, 2003.

Maslach, Christina and Michael P. Leiter. *The Truth about Burnout: How Organizations Cause Personal Stress and What to Do about It.* San Francisco: Jossey-Bass, 1997.

Merton, Thomas. *New Seeds of Contemplation.* New York: New Directions Publishing, 1962; *Contemplative Prayer.* New York: Image Books, 1971.

Miller, Alice. *The Drama of the Gifted Child: The Search for the True Self.* New York: Basic Books, 1997.

Moore, Robert and Douglass Gillette, *King, Warrior, Magician, Lover: Rediscovering the Archetypes of the Mature Masculine* (New York: HarperCollins, 1990).

Nepo, Mark. *Inside the Miracle: Enduring Suffering, Approaching Wholeness.* Louisville, Colorado: Sounds True, 2015.

Nouwen, Henri. *The Wounded Healer.* New York: Doubleday, 1979.

Nouwen, Henri, *The Return of the Prodigal Son: A Story of Homecoming* (New York: Doubleday, 1992).

Nouwen, Henri, *Spiritual Formation: Following of the Movements of the Spirit* (New York: HarperCollins, 2010).

O'Brien, Tim. *The Things They Carried.* New York: Broadway Books, 1990.

Ofri, Danielle. *What Doctors Feel: How Emotions Affect the Practice of Medicine.* Boston, Massachusetts: Beacon Press, 2013.

Quinones, Sam. *Dreamland: The True Tale of America's Opiate Epidemic*. New York: Bloomsbury Press, 2016.

Rohr, Richard. *Adam's Return: The Five Promises of Male Initiation*. New York: The Crossroad Publishing Co., 2004; *The Divine Dance*. New Kensington, Pennsylvania: Whitaker House, 2016; *Everything Belongs: The Gift of Contemplative Prayer*. New York: The Crossroad Publishing Co., 2003; *Falling Upward: A Spirituality for the Two Halves of Life*. San Francisco, California: Jossey-Bass, 2011; *Immortal Diamond: The Search for Our True Self*. San Francisco, California: Jossey-Bass, 2013; *Things Hidden: Scripture as Spirituality*. Cincinnati, Ohio: Franciscan Media, 2008.

Ryken, Leland, ed. *The Christian Imagination: The Practice of Faith Literature and Writing*. New York: Waterbrook Multnomah (Penguin Random House), 2002.

Ryken, Philip, *Art for God's Sake: A Call to Recover the Arts*. Phillipsburg, New Jersey: P&R Publishing Co., 2006.

Sandum, David *I'll Run Till the Sun Goes Down: A Memoir about Depression and Discovering Art*. Boulder, Colorado: Sandra Jonas Publishing House, 2016.

Schneider, Pat. *How the Light Gets In: Writing as a Spiritual Practice*. New York: Oxford University Press, 2013.

Seerveld, Calvin. *Rainbows for the Fallen World*. Toronto: Tuppence Press, 1980.

St John of the Cross, *Dark Night of the Soul* (New York: Dover 2003)

Treier, Daniel J., Mark Husbands, Roger Lundin, eds. *The Beauty of God: Theology and the Arts*. Downers Grove, Illinois: InterVarsity Press, 2007.

W., Bill. *Twelve Steps and Twelve Traditions*. New York: Alcoholics Anonymous World Services, 1981.